STAND UP STRAIGHT

*personal recollections
about scoliosis by the people
who live with it*

Iris Halberstam-Mickel

Medical Introduction by
L. Carl Samberg, M.D.
Orthopedic Surgeon

KENDALL/HUNT PUBLISHING COMPANY
2460 Kerper Boulevard   P.O. Box 539   Dubuque, Iowa 52004-0539

TO THE READER

The names of the people interviewed have been changed to protect their privacy. The stories are true recollections. This book is not intended as a substitute for consulting with your physician. Proper treatment of scoliosis requires a doctor's supervision.

MELVINDALE PUBLIC LIBRAR
18650 ALLEN RD.
MELVINDALE, MI 48122
381-8677

Cover design and drawings on pages 4, 5, 104, 106 and 107 by Robert Graves-Wesolosky.

Copyright © 1989 by Iris J. Mickel

Library of Congress Catalog Card Number: 88-84108

ISBN 0-8403-5223-9

All rights reserved. No part of this publication may be reproduced, stored in a retrieval system, or transmitted, in any form or by any means, electronic, mechanical, photocopying, recording, or otherwise, without the prior written permission of the copyright owner.

Printed in the United States of America
10 9 8 7 6 5 4 3 2 1

*To my children, Shari, Jodi, and Amy . . .
my reasons.*

Contents

Acknowledgments	vii
Preface	ix
Foreword	xi

Part I Medical Introduction—*L. Carl Samberg, M.D.* **1**

Chapter 1. Scoliosis: The Definition and Nature of the Problem	3
Chapter 2. Natural History of "Untreated" Scoliosis	8
Chapter 3. Don't Forget the Adult	11
Chapter 4. Yet Unanswered Questions	13
Chapter 5. Progress in the Treatment of Scoliosis	14
Chapter 6. The Most Frequently Asked Questions about Scoliosis . . . Answered!	17

Part II Interviews **21**

Chapter 1. Stand Up Straight! Adults Who Have Had Two Surgeries, One as a Child and One as an Adult	23
Natalie	24
Katherine	29
Caroline	32
Marlene	34
Chapter 2. It Could Be Worse! Living with Pain. Adults Who Have Had Treatment Other than Surgery	37
Miles	38
Cora	40
Freida	41
Martha	43

Frank	44
Eli	46
Imogene	48
Marge	50
Shirley	51
Bonnie	53
Cassie	55

Chapter 3. Accentuating the Positive! Adults Who Have Had Surgery as Children — 58

Sharon	59
Brenda	61
Dorene	62
Elaine	63
Sylvia	64
Marion	65

Chapter 4. Learning to Live with It—Or Is There Life After Scoliosis? Men and Women Choosing to Have Surgery as Adults — 67

Liz	68
Jessica	70
Jane	72
Louise	73
Leslie	76
Bob	78
Pamela	80
Patricia	82
Jerry	84
Melissa	86
Margaret-Ann	87
Kim	89

Chapter 5. I Married My Wife for Her Curves! The Spouses Respond — 91

Chapter 6. Update . . . Scoliosis: A Discussion — 94

Part III Getting It Straight — 101

Chapter 1. How to Look for a Spinal Deformity — 103

Chapter 2. Postural Exercises for Scoliosis — 105

Chapter 3. Glossary of Scoliosis Terms — 108

Chapter 4. Reference List of Recommended Reading — 112

Acknowledgments

I wrote this book for people who have endured scoliosis in silence. I wrote it for those still suffering silently, and for their families who have no place to turn with their questions. I wrote this book for future generations with the hope that the feelings expressed, within, will help make living with scoliosis easier.

To my husband Harold, my wonderful family, and dear friends who never once questioned or doubted my ability to complete this work, thank you! To my doctor and co-author, L. Carl Samberg, M.D., thank you for helping me dig beneath the surface and sort out many thoughts and feelings. Your encouragement through some very rough moments and your faith in our ability to make it through, made a concept materialize.

I wish to sincerely thank the following people for their editorial comments, helping me to locate reference materials, use equipment, offer advice and suggestions, review rough drafts, and help me to evaluate ideas: Carl D. Brenner, Certified Prosthetist and Orthotist; Ann Chowdhury; Richard Curtis, Literary Agent; the late Michael J. Halberstam, M.D.; Shirlee Rose-Iden; Frank C. Kava, Physical Therapist; Alvin B. Michaels, M.D.; Philip S. Peven, M.D.; Jerry H. Rosenberg, M.D.; Lori Strager; and D. Eugene Thompson, M.D. Finally, a very special thanks to Robert Graves-Wesolosky for the graphic concepts.

My most sincere thanks to the people who were interviewed and who shared their special thoughts, stories and experiences. Their willingness to bring out into the open so many well kept secrets is most certain to help others with scoliosis.

The following poem was written by Diana Ortopan, following her spinal fusion. It is a beautiful and inspiring message for anyone contemplating surgery or having gone through a spinal fusion. Poetry has always been an important part of her life. Diane was born on July 16, 1943 and died on July 2, 1984.

ONE CHRISTMAS

Once in a forest
stood a tiny pine tree
with a twisted trunk,
only four foot three.
Families were searching
as Christmas was near
for the perfect pine
as they did each year.
"I'll never be chosen,"
cried the little tree.
"I'll never wear tinsel
for all to see."
"You shouldn't be crying,"
chirped a nearby jay.
"it's Christmas time,
and you should be gay."
"Jesus didn't have tinsel
and colored light
when he came to us
on that special night."
And so on Christmas Eve
it snowed and snowed
while the tiny pine slept
and the forest glowed.
Slowly, as if in a dream,
on that snowy night
the twisted tree turned
first left, then right.
And when in the morning
the pine tree woke,
he stood tall and straight
in a white snowy cloak.

Preface

By
Barbara M. Shulman, President
The Scoliosis Association, Inc.

Scoliosis is not merely a word or a definition. It is first and foremost a condition that, if one has it, it must be lived with on a daily basis. Scoliosis requires adjustments by patient, family, friends and physician in order to successfully adapt to life with it. It is for this very reason—successful adaptation—that the Scoliosis Association, Inc. came into being. It is through this organization and its chapters and international affiliates that we attempt to help individuals make a positive adjustment to living with scoliosis.

There is inestimable value in communicating with others who "have been there." We, the members of the Scoliosis Association, are kindred spirits who can empathize with those who seek our assistance. Many, just like the readers of this book, initially come to us knowing little about scoliosis. Through exposure to correct information, they become comfortable with their situation and are then able to start making adjustments and decisions about their scoliosis. How one adjusts to the knowledge gained depends on many factors. Individual attitude is the result of environment—family and social attitudes with which we all interrelate. Positive and outgoing personality traits develop as a result of encouraging, supportive attitudes of family members and friends. The converse can often result in a negative personal image.

Dr. Samberg and Ms. Mickel have attempted in *Stand Up Straight!* to put scoliosis into perspective by giving an overview of the condition and relating stories as told to Ms. Mickel by other scoliotics. Many of those interviewed relate incidents that represent the existing modalities of treatment at the time of their experiences. It is through insight gained during their treatment that both the medical and lay communities benefited. The future is always built on the past.

The "state of the art" of treating scoliosis has changed greatly over the years. One thing still remains. Scoliosis is a condition to which one must adjust. Research is ongoing; answers are falling into place; but in the meantime, we do not have to "suffer in silence." Scoliosis can be successfully treated. Life can and will go on. To quote one of the interviewees, "You have every right to enjoy the good things in life. You deserve those things too."

The message of the Scoliosis Association, Inc. and this book is that "scoliosis doesn't make you an invalid in any way. It doesn't mean you can do things better (you may try harder) than anyone else, but you have every reason to feel that you are every bit as good as everyone else."

The need for a book of this nature has long been obvious to people afflicted with scoliosis. They search for references and materials about others similarly afflicted. This has been frequently a futile search. Here in one volume, is an explanation of scoliosis and a cross section of personal experiences which may help others to make a positive adjustment to scoliosis.

Stand Up Straight! should help the Scoliosis Association and its chapters reach one of its prime goals—that of helping people to adjust in a positive manner and to develop an ability to cope with their diverse and individual scoliosis problems.

Foreword

DOCTOR'S REPORT: January 6, 1984

PATIENT: Iris Mickel   **DOCTOR:** L. Carl Samberg, M.D.

AGE: 39 years 5 months

Last films in October, 1981, demonstrated a double major curve pattern with a right thoracic curve pattern measured from T3 through T12 at 73 degrees and an associated left lumbar scoliosis of 80 degrees from T12 through L5. Overall balance of the spine was quite good at that time with the plumb line dropped from the base of the neck falling in the midline. In review of films dating back to October, 1977, suggest that there has been absolutely no change in the curve over that period of time. As we had discussed, the absence of continuing curve progression suggested at least, at last study, that a surgical procedure was not absolutely indicated. (See figure 1.)

I am the victim of scoliosis. This condition, which is the side-to-side curvature of the spine, has no known cause, no known cure, and is considered a serious orthopedic problem facing children today.

In 1957 I had a spinal fusion, whereby bone was grafted from my left leg and placed along the major curve on my spine, fusing approximately six vertebrae making a solid mass of bone. This procedure was done to stop the progression of the curve in the major curve area.

In the thirty or more years since the actual discovery and treatment of my scoliosis, I have been poked, researched, exercised and examined—and I still live with a severe spinal deformity.

I have personally lived through the trauma of having scoliosis. With more than 30 years of treatment behind me, finally these bits and pieces of memories have come together into some meaningful form. Looking back, I did fine. I missed a lot of socialization during the ages of 12 to

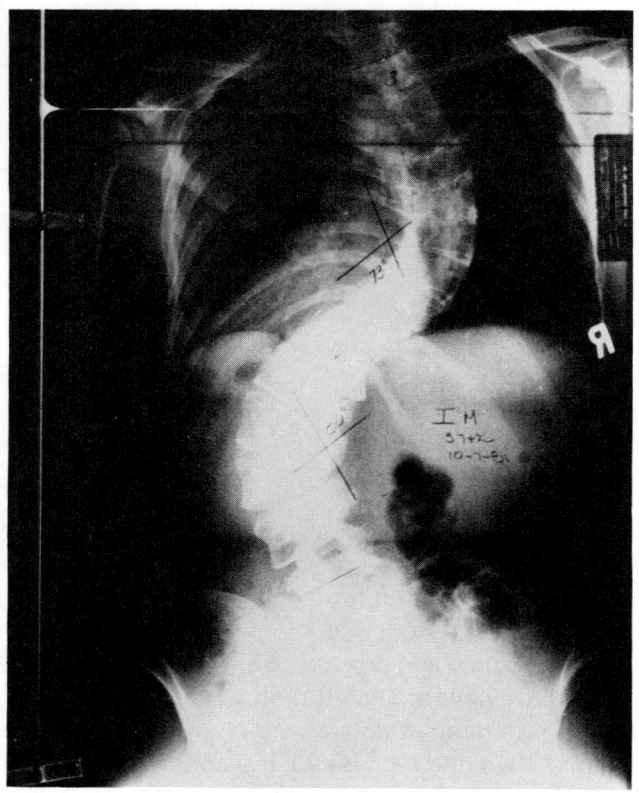

Figure 1. SCOLIOSIS is a spinal deformity that, when left to progress, could cause heart and lung damage, changes in physical appearance, pain, and sometimes early death.

14, giving me a social lag. During my surgery and the post-operative period of six months lying flat on my back with a full body cast, I managed to keep busy with school assignments from an inservice teacher. Friends and family came to visit often, but they were all busy enjoying school friendships, parties, and their own personal activities. I didn't fully recognize the extent of how much I was bothered by these repressed feelings from my childhood until my daughter, Shari, at the age of 10½ began to show visible signs of having scoliosis. That is, she had one shoulder higher than the other, a protruding right shoulder blade, and right rib rotation.

That nasty curve! Why wasn't I forewarned that my children could have this same condition? Flashes of memories from my childhood kept appearing in my mind. This time, anger motivated me to make a change. I took Shari to our pediatrician who tried to comfort me by saying, "Don't be alarmed, girls often develop faster on one side than the other." Why is this happening to me, I thought. Twenty-five years later, and attitudes remain the same? There must be someone to share this with, someone who has had a similar experience.

Determined to find others with whom to share experiences, I wrote a short meeting notice which I submitted to our local newspaper. The notice invited interested families to get together at an elementary school to informally discuss their feelings about scoliosis. I then contacted an orthopedic surgeon, a pediatrician, and a leader in a service group to be the guest speakers and offer a question and answer session on the subject of scoliosis. Shirlee Iden, a writer for the *Southfield Observer Eccentric,* ran the notice about the meeting. Forty people attended that first gathering on December 6, 1976. The people who attended came for a variety of reasons, but mostly to have their questions about scoliosis answered. A real purpose developed from this meeting. That purpose was to promote an early detection program in Michigan to screen children in the schools for scoliosis and related spinal deformities, and to give families and patients support by providing programs and services. These meetings continued until March of 1977 when we joined with The Scoliosis Association, Inc. becoming their second chapter.

Attitudes are changing, information is being made available and questions are now being answered. Too many people lived with scoliosis in pain and needless discomfort. Too many people lived with scoliosis with unanswered questions. In order to come to peace with oneself, to understand the limitations one has, and to learn to live and cope with the deformity, feelings must be confronted.

The people who have been interviewed in the chapters to follow recall their most private emotions and reflect upon their past experiences to bring about a meaningful picture of scoliosis. In order to improve upon treatment, we must examine the past and allow those individuals who have been a part of that treatment to talk. The treatment from the past has had an emotional and psychological impact on the individuals interviewed. The outcome of the interviews reflect a change in attitude about treatment and surgery from the 1920's to the 1980's. We begin with an "I'm angry" attitude from the past to an "I'm so happy" reflection from current treatment.

PART I
Medical Introduction

L. Carl Samberg, M.D.

CHAPTER 1

SCOLIOSIS: The Definition and Nature of the Problem

Scoliosis is defined as a lateral-rotatory curvature of the spine and is the most common of spinal deformities. Viewed from the side, the spine has certain curvatures, which are normal and essential to the maintenance of upright posture. These are cervical lordosis, thoracic kyphosis and lumbar lordosis. Those curves are only of concern when excessive or exaggerated. The spine when viewed from behind should be perfectly straight and in good balance standing upright over the pelvic base. Any deviation from that straight spine is called scoliosis. (See figure 2 and 3.)

Spine deformity such as scoliosis must be regarded as a symptom rather than a disease, since there are many causes. Scoliosis is classified according to definitive or theoretical cause as being congenital (born with); secondary to neuromuscular disease (as in Poliomyelitis and other paralytic disorders); related to certain other conditions affecting the spine such as arthritis, neurofibromatosis and connective tissue disorders; postural, such as that associated with leg length discrepancies and the largest classifed group is known as idiopathic. Idiopathic means cause unknown.

Though scoliosis is by no means a new problem, only recently have prevalence studies received more than passing attention. From data obtained through school screening programs in the past decade has come the realization that scoliosis is more prevalent than previously suspected. Males were more frequently involved than heretofore reported. Many curves of minor magnitude exist and progression of those curves is by no means universal.

If age 16 is used as a point of study, approximately 2–3 percent of the population will have scoliosis measuring in excess of 10°. With small curves, the sex ratio is equal—males to females—that is in curves of less than 10°. As children grow, progression is much more likely in girls than boys, and approximately 2% will require some aggressive treatment; that is, more than observation alone. All curves discovered need to be followed, since absolute clues as to which curves will progress and which

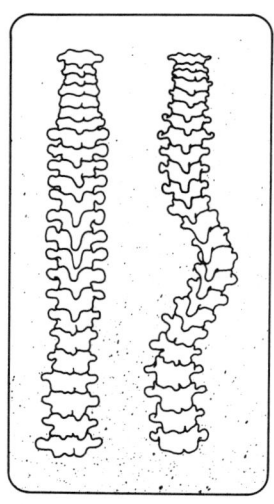

Figure 2. A normal spine (left).
Figure 3. A scoliotic spine (right).

will not are yet lacking. The risk of progression depends on the patient's age and degree of curvature, with incidence equal in young patients with mild curves and female predominance in older patients with advancing curves. Curve progression typically occurs during the adolescent growth spurt.

Idiopathic means cause unknown. Much study is currently being done with regard to possible causes and certain information exists to implicate it as an inherited condition. Idiopathic scoliosis accounts for approximately 80% of all cases of scoliosis. Many of those who, in the past, attributed their curvatures to either injury or polio, did in fact, have idiopathic scoliosis.

There is a large body of evidence that suggests that abnormalities in the central nervous system may play a role in causing idiopathic scoliosis. It is possible that certain sub-clinical abnormalities of the central nervous system represent the primary problem in idiopathic scoliosis.

Curve patterns are named for the area of the spine in which they occur. The spine is anatomically divided into four major regions: cervical or neck area; thoracic, which is associated with the rib cage; lumbar, which is related to the abdominal area; and sacral or base of the spine. A curve existing in the thoracic region is, therefore, termed a thoracic curve; those in the lumbar area are called lumbar curves, and so on. Some curves are multiple and flow from one area to another, hence the term double curve or "S" curve. Those curves which extend from one area into another are

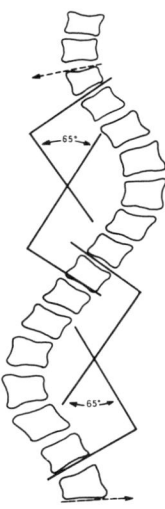

Figure 4. Demonstration of Cobb Method of curve measurement.

named for both regions; for example, thoracolumbar curve with its middle at the junction of the thoracic and lumbar section of the spine.

Over the years, scoliosis was, to some degree, discovered—not studied—and allowed to take its course without any treatment being rendered. Any scientific measure of the initial curve or of its ultimate severity was non-existent. Curves were simply viewed as being: mild, severe, bad or worse. Careful observation and an accurate method of measurement has allowed for meaningful follow-up of curves. No longer does progression go unnoticed, nor are the curves of greater magnitude ignored. Serial study of curves by comparative measurements allows that proper treatment can be given to each patient and each spinal curvature.

X-ray evaluation of curves at appropriate intervals are now carefully measured and compared with prior studies of that same patient. Any curve progression can then be readily detected and dealt with. It is suggested that a single x-ray exposure is all that is needed to determine if a scoliotic curve exists. The patient should stand with equal weight on each foot, in a relaxed, upright position. In most instances, enough of the spine can be demonstrated on a 14 × 17 film to determine the existence of a scoliotic deformity. If there is no evidence of scoliosis on the initial erect film, no further x-rays are required. When additional films are needed, several techniques can reduce the radiation dosage to the child, including the use of fast, rare earth screen film combinations, compensating filters and shielding.

The standard method of measure adopted by the Scoliosis Research Society for determining the size of a curve is the Cobb method of measurement. Lines are drawn along the superior and inferior end plates of the vertebral bodies at each end of the curve. Those end vertebra are the last ones that are tilted into the concavity of a particular curve. The angle of intersection formed by perpendiculars to those lines determines the scoliotic angle. It is important that all subsequent films be measured in a similar fashion. This allows comparison of films and recording of what is happening to the curve. Any curve progression can then be readily detected and dealt with. (See figure 4.)

The age at which a curve is detected, and therefore presumed to begin, determines whether it is called *infantile* (birth to 3 years), *juvenile* (3 years to puberty), or *adolescent* (from puberty through the end of growth) scoliosis. Not all curves progress, but recent studies have suggested that there are certain factors which may be important in terms of determining which are most likely to take a progressive course. Scoliosis generally begins in youth and is intimately associated with growth and development. Because most methods of treatment are aimed at preventing progression, information regarding growth and maturation patterns is needed. Studies in Scandinavia and North America suggest that teenage girls and boys with scoliosis are significantly taller at given chronologic ages. Late skeletal and sexual development also has seemed to be a characteristic of that group of children, and particularly for those girls with larger curves. Such delay in skeletal maturation may be significant, since the period of adolescence is extended, prolonging the risk of curve progression to severity by delaying stabilization of the scoliotic spine. Because the delay is greater in girls with larger curves, skeletal and sexual immaturity must be considered risk signs for curve progression. The younger the child at initial detection of the curve, the greater is the chance for serious curve progression.

With increasing age, there is a decreasing risk of progression. The curve detected in a girl prior to the onset of menstrual periods has a much greater chance of progression (66%) than one detected postmenarchy (33%). The larger the initial curvature detected, the greater is the chance of progression.

Some curves are completely correctable with side bending and are called non-structural or functional curves. They tend not to progress while those structural or more fixed curves stand a greater chance of progression. Flexible curves often exist along with structural curves and are the result of the body's attempt to compensate or balance the spine in which the fixed curve exists. Once the main curve is corrected, there is no longer any need for the compensatory curve and it spontaneously disappears. Curves in the thoracic region in excess of 40° at discovery in a yet skeletally immature child have a better than 70 percent chance of progressing. Those that exceed 30° have an even chance of increasing during the yet remaining period of growth. With the beginning of puberty and its associated rapid growth spurt, those curves destined to progress may do so significantly during the years of remaining growth. Again, however, it must be emphasized that *not all curves do progress*. Lacking additional specifics in each instance, it is imperative that *all* be followed.

CHAPTER 2
Natural History of "Untreated" Scoliosis

Why treat scoliosis? What happens to the patient with scoliosis who is not treated? These are questions which can only be answered by a careful analysis of the natural history of untreated scoliosis—through a look into the past.

Major myths have been promulgated which have over the years, to some degree, limited progress in the field of scoliosis treatment. Spinal deformities were once regarded as self-limiting conditions in childhood, terminating at the completion of growth, and beyond that point, not worthy of further consideration. The group of adults with scoliosis have, as a result, been neglected and hidden. Even when scoliosis was recognized in adults, it was held that not much could be done about it and was, perhaps, better left without attention. Treatment often resulted in dismal failure, and certain social stigmata were at least sensed by those who recognized that they had scoliosis.

Studies of the natural history of untreated scoliosis over the past few decades have exploded some of those myths, and have led to a more scholarly approach to treatment and a better understanding of the need for treatment.

Adulthood with regard to spinal maturity cannot be viewed arbitrarily on the basis of age. An adult is a person who has ceased to grow and in whom all growth centers are closed precluding any additional growth. This can vary in people between 18 and 25 years, generally occurring later in men than in women.

Scoliosis in an untreated adult may behave in three ways. First, it may become stable at skeletal maturity and never progress at all. Secondly, it may progress slowly throughout the life of the individual. Or, thirdly, it may remain relatively stable or static in early adult life, only to worsen with the degenerative processes and bone softening of later life.

To a great degree, the ultimate course of scoliosis in the adult depends upon the curve type and magnitude which exists in a given individual at the moment of completion of growth. To be sure, it can no longer be said that the curve which exists at skeletal maturity, in all cases, is the curve which will exist throughout the life of that person and, therefore, deserves no further consideration. This major myth has been exploded.

It is now generally agreed that those curves which exist in excess of 50° at skeletal maturity will almost certainly tend to progress. Lesser curves, and certainly those of less than 30°, which are well compensated, remain stable throughout life. Those curves, however, which are located in the lumbar spine, perhaps by virtue of their lacking the support of the rib cage, tend to be more at risk of progression at the same magnitude. The problem, then, is that one must virtually speculate about what will be the course of those curves which fall between 25° and 50°.

It is now obvious to those who treat scoliosis that, adequately treated during adolescence, balanced curves of less than 25° rarely progress and significant problems do not occur during adult life. If balance has not been achieved by completion of growth, however, then increasing scoliosis continues with some frequency, even in those small curves. The ideal situation, then, is a small curve in good balance. That is exactly the aim of all treatment in pre-adult years.

In general, thoracolumbar and lumbar curves tend more toward progression. There is a much higher incidence of back pain in those persons than in those with well-balanced curves of similar magnitude in the thoracic spine. Patients with double major patterns in good balance also tend to do relatively well, at least until later years, with back pain intervening only with serious degenerative processes.

Large thoracic curves, when they progress, can lead to increasing compromise of pulmonary function producing a decrease in exercise tolerance and shortness of breath. These problems especially develop in situations in which there also exists serious kyphosis or roundback deformities. Both the scoliosis kyphotic deformities tend to progress as a result of osteoporosis or bone softening with aging.

Adult patients generally present themselves to a physician because they have pain or are concerned with what they perceive as an increasing cosmetic deformity. Either the curve and deformity have actually changed, or they have for some reason become less able to see themselves as they once did. Pain can lead to incapacity in work or play, and self-image problems may impose definite changes in lifestyles.

Back pain has been estimated to be an occurring entity, at least one time, for over 80 percent of us. There may be a slightly higher incidence or more frequent occurrence in those with scoliosis. This is certainly true in those with large lumbar and thoraco-lumbar curves.

The patterns of pain in those with scoliosis are not dissimilar to those seen in non-scoliotic patients with degenerative back changes. Bracing support and other conservative measures such as exercises and pain medication generally solve these problems, with a need for more involved forms of treatment being by no means universal for those with scoliosis. Surgery should in no way then be considered the solution to all scoliosis in adults. There must, instead, be very specific reasons for surgery. One cannot generalize about those in a text such as this. Specifics as to who will require an operation for their scoliosis, which operation should be done, and so on, can only be given by one's treating physician after careful evaluation and thoughtful consideration of that patient and his/her unique problems.

Radiographs or x-rays have not been well protected and saved over the years. But, where they are available, they are invaluable in determining whether there has or has not been progression of a particular scoliotic curve. Patients may also note changes in height over a period of years, which loss can be an indication of curve progression. Similarly, one's appreciation that a rib prominence has increased in size may be a clue to a developing curve progression.

Cardiopulmonary compromise leading to extreme difficulties with breathing and heart failure can develop in severe curves with progression when left untreated. Generally, no significant compromise exists in curves of less than 60° or 70°, and then only in thoracic curves with major rib deformation. Certainly not all, and in fact few with scoliosis die young, but *all* must be followed so that curve progression does not go undetected and untreated increasing that threat.

Body image is of personal concern to all. Cosmesis is not an unimportant factor in scoliosis. Complaints of pain and disability can often times be expanded in the mind of the patient by dissatisfaction with his physical appearance. An attempt to be as objective as possible about a specific complaint in each patient is important for both physician and patient.

What can be said, then, about the natural history of scoliosis is that certain curves tend to progress; that scoliosis is not necessarily static in adult life; and that adults do require long-term follow-up. Such problems as pain, cosmetic disfigurement, breathing difficulties and disability are best avoided by an aggressive approach to the child with scoliosis and through long-term follow-up in all patients with scoliosis. Progress in treatment can only come about when we know what has happened in the past and have evaluated how successful prior treatment has been. *Since some curves in some patients do progress, it is incumbent upon us to follow all with frequency.* Armed with such information about what a particular curve has done and what might be expected, allows a treatment program to be rationally planned.

CHAPTER **3**

Don't Forget the Adult

Scoliosis has, in the past, been generally considered a problem of adolescents. Though we now recognize that the detection of scoliosis and its proper treatment at that age is the answer to most problems, there are adult patients who were not fortunate enough to have their scoliosis detected and treated early.

Educational material made more generally available to adults through the school screening of their children has allowed those older patients afflicted with scoliosis to express their concerns and/or seek appropriate treatment.

Considerations such as pain, difficulty with breathing and cosmetic appearance all contribute to the worries of daily life for adults with scoliosis.

What is the prognosis for the adult scoliosis patient? What are the physical and emotional needs of an adult who must carry a curved spine throughout life? The answers to these and other questions are developing as more and more of these questions are being addressed by treating physicians and support groups. Scoliosis in adults does progress, and progression when it occurs is a definite indication for surgical stabilization when the individual's general health allows such a procedure. Breathing problems and pain, though by no means universally occurring in scoliosis patients, are generally considered reasons for surgical intervention.

In recent years, increasing safety in the performance of surgical procedures in adults has made such treatment for some an appropriate course. An adult is defined as an individual who has completed growth. Scoliosis in an adult may behave in three ways depending on such factors as curve size, location and intrinsic flexibility. The curve may stabilize and no longer progress beyond skeletal maturity. It may slowly become more severe or worsen or it may not progress early in life only to become more severe with aging and the degenerative change in later decades beyond the 5th or 6th.

Aside from these considerations, the study of the psycho-social adaptation of scoliosis in patients is important. Scoliosis patients do have more difficulty finding employment; poor body image often leads to difficulties in entering into social and marriage situations, as well as influencing recreational and hobby interests.

It is to the solution of these types of problems that local support groups affiliated with The Scoliosis Association, Inc. can best be addressed. No longer should patients with scoliosis consider themselves handicapped, for scoliosis is for most a treatable condition. Physicians and those lay support groups must convince employers that persons with scoliosis can and do work well, are liked by others, make wonderful parents and are truly born in the *image of God*. Those who have gone before and experienced the growing pains of progress in scoliosis (and many of those stories are reflected in the interviews portrayed in this text) should "Stand Up Straight" and in fact *with pride,* "Stand Tall" for you have given much to the future of our children.

CHAPTER 4
Yet Unanswered Questions

The cause of scoliosis remains a complex mystery. Voluminous literature related to possible etiologic factors lead us to conclude that it is a multifactoral problem. In an attempt to correlate efforts in the endless pursuit of the cause, the Scoliosis Research Society, in 1982, initiated what it hopes will be an ongoing international and annual review of present efforts at discovery. (Only fitting was the keynote introduction to that endeavor in memory of Dr. Paul Harrington, who contributed so much to our present knowledge of scoliosis.)

In the papers that followed, many meaningful theses were put forth. Investigation will continue until one day the pieces of the puzzle will fit together and then, possibly, hopefully, the need for the trying of difficult treatment measures of today will be no more.

Work is being done in the study of growth factors, skeletal maturity, chemical variations, genetic considerations, balance and righting reactions, mechanical and structural factors and constant review of the natural history of scoliosis patients.

CHAPTER 5
Progress in the Treatment of Scoliosis

In 1974, Dr. Robert Winter, a now renowned scoliosis surgeon, delivered an important message to the Scoliosis Research Society in his presidential address. That message was by way of a challenge to us all to wisely use from the past and with forward vision to apply principles learned through the careful follow-up of those previously treated to plan for the next era in scoliosis management.

Following the first successful spine fusion in 1911 the surgical management of scoliosis has been advanced by such visionary developers as Cobb, Risser and Moe in the improvement of surgical techniques for fusion of the spine. Instrumentation added to these techniques by Harrington, Dwyer and many others has allowed even adult scoliosis patients to derive good results with resolution of their problems. Distortion of the spine is not static at skeletal maturity but often advancing and requiring stabilization if problems with pain, increasing deformity and potential cardiorespiratory difficulties ensue. No longer should things be let go until surgery is needed. Scoliosis is best treated before the end of growth. The key to successful treatment is early detection of a small problem. Non-operative treatment modalities can then be applied to prevent progression.

The early detection of scoliosis has without question been aided by school screening programs. Beginning with the early screening programs for scoliosis and other orthopedic diseases in Delaware in the early 1960's and through the development of many programs throughout the United States and the world much has been learned about the incidence of scoliosis among school-age children. The early detection of spine deformities has been proven to be effective in bringing to treating physicians both those early cases in which treatment can be most effective and also a wealth of information about the natural history and anticipated course of those discovered curves. For many, school screening has truly been as advertised, "a thirty second wise investment for a lifetime of dividends."

The management of patients with scoliosis is constantly changing, and change it must, if any progress is to be made. The treatment of scoliosis at any age in the patient's life is aimed at preventing curve progression. In the growing period when a progressive curve is recognized, an aggressive treatment program must be undertaken. The older the child and the less spinal growth that is anticipated, the more conservative the treatment approach can be. If continued spinal growth is anticipated, any curve of more than 10 degrees is allowed to progress at least 10 degrees before any treatment is initiated. Curves over 20 degrees are generally watched more carefully and less curve progression is required to initiate treatment. Larger curves, that is greater than 30 degrees, are generally, initially braced to prevent progression. Over the years, numerous braces have been advocated for the management of scoliosis. The Milwaukee brace developed by Drs. Blount and Schmidt remains the benchmark by which all others must be measured. The goal of bracing is to prevent curve progression and improvement in the curve is generally not expected. Measurements at the end of treatment may show some improvement. Long term maintenance of that correction is generally not retained. More recently, curves in the lower back have been managed with so-called low profile braces which are more cosmetically acceptable and as effective for those low curves. The choice of brace type, however, is not arbitrary and the appropriate brace for a curve can only be determined by the treating physician. Electrical stimulation in the management of spinal curvatures has been advocated over the past 15 years. Initially implanted electrodes were used to obtain temporary correction. These required a surgical procedure of some magnitude and long term results have not been as good as initially anticipated. Surface electrodes, though initially suggesting great promise, have also proved discouraging. The late results of electrical stimulation do not appear to have altered significantly the natural history of idiopathic scoliosis.

In those patients in whom so-called conservative techniques have failed, the surgical approach is indicated. It must be kept in mind that the purpose of any surgical procedure for scoliosis is to obtain a solid fusion and thereby prevent further curve progression.

Advances in anesthesia and surgical technique have greatly minimized the risks involved in surgical management. The patients once told nothing could be done, are now offered a chance at an improved future. The use of autologous blood transfusion during surgery and other measures which minimize blood loss have significantly added to safety.

Once a surgical course is decided upon, it is important to select the proper surgical procedure. The operation is called a spinal fusion and its purpose is to prevent further curve progression. Spinal cord monitoring further adds to the safety of the procedure. The surgeon must carefully plan which part of the spine is to be fused taking into consideration curve pattern and overall spine balance and stability.

The last decade has seen an explosion of instrumentation aimed at obtaining greater curve correction and greater post operative stability making post operative casting less necessary. The Harrington instrumentation system was the first effective instrumentation developed to correct scoliotic curvature. It remains the *gold standard* and all other systems must be measured by it. Variations on that same theme over time have included the Drummond system combining Harrington with Luque rod and spinous process wiring and double distraction hook instrumentation with the Harrington rod, the so-called Bobechko procedure. Segmental fixation advocated by Eduardo Luque and anterior instrumentation with Dwyer or Zielke systems all can be offered to patients with scoliosis. The choice of these procedures is best left to the surgeon who carefully weighs the appropriateness of a particular instrumentation system for each patient and his or her particular curve problem. Various techniques should be discussed with the surgeon prior to deciding on technique.

It is incumbent upon those of us who treat scoliosis as well as upon those of us who have scoliosis that we better our world. We must see what we have done, critically analyze the results of applied therapies and make changes where needed. Someone once said that "if you could invent a better mousetrap the world would beat a path to your door." Many new mousetraps have been developed for the management of scoliosis and paths have been beaten. We must remember that for something to be worthy of consideration in life it must be new and it must be better. Some of the developments such as electrical stimulation of muscles to correct scoliosis and the development of new braces have yet to be proven over time. They certainly are promising and reflect "the changing state of the art." Surgical techniques must be judged based not on immediate results with regard to curve correction but on the lasting ability to solve each patient's problem and not contribute to long-term difficulties.

CHAPTER **6**

The Most Frequently Asked Questions . . . Answered By: L. Carl Samberg, M.D.

Statement: To answer a question, one always draws upon the current body of knowledge relative to a particular problem. Then one presents to the questioner his interpretation of that body of knowledge as it relates to the inquiry. Specific questions relative to your scoliosis are best answered by the physician caring for you. Some generalizations relative to what seem frequently asked questions are listed in the following.

1. *What will happen to the Harrington Rod several years down the road? Should I have it removed?*

   ANSWER: In general, once a spinal fusion becomes solid, the Harrington Rod presents no problem. In the event that no difficulties do develop, there is generally no reason to remove the rod. Any surgical procedure must have an absolute indication and carries with it certain risks. Those risks are not warranted simply for the removal of a rod unless specific problems related to that rod ensue.

2. *What are the chances of my present spinal fusion causing me problems 10 or 20 years from now?*

   ANSWER: The record of patients treated with spinal fusion 20 years ago would suggest that in instances where a good solid spinal fusion has been achieved, serious problems associated with scoliosis have been obviated. Barring instances of rod fracture or inadequate fusion, patients generally do well and have little chance of serious difficulty.

3. *Will one surgery for scoliosis end the problem of continual curving?*

   ANSWER: Each curve has its own characteristics. Each patient's curve is distinctly different from others and approaches to the surgical management of scoliosis do even to this date differ from one treating surgeon to another. Though one surgical procedure generally resolves all problems, it may not, in a specific instance, prevent curvature of the spine above and/or below an area fused.

4. *Am I more susceptible to injury to my back from a fall now that I have had a spinal fusion?*

   ANSWER: The term spinal fusion does imply stiffness and patients with spinal fusion do lose some flexibility in the spine which is a protective mechanism against injury. Though generally they are no more susceptible to injury than others, certain types of activity might best be avoided. Those include contact sports and participation in diving and tumbling activities.

5. *How long does it take for a spinal fusion to become a solid mass of bone?*

   ANSWER: Though generally by one year spinal fusions are solid enough to allow a return to near normal life styles, the fusion mass probably is not completely solid for approximately 2 to 2½ years, and during that time risk laden athletic activities should be avoided.

6. *When are you considered too old for a spinal fusion?*

   ANSWER: One is perhaps never too old for a spinal fusion, provided his/her general physical condition is such that risks related to the surgical procedure are not undue and the chances of procuring a good fusion are satisfactory.

7. *How soon after scoliosis surgery can I consider getting pregnant?*

   ANSWER: Generally it is best to avoid mechanical stress which pregnancy might produce upon the spinal fusion until the fusion mass is solid at approximately two years post surgery.

8. *Will having children cause problems with the fusion or interfere with the Harrington Rod:*

   ANSWER: There is absolutely no evidence that pregnancy, child bearing and delivery cause any problem with the fusion or interfere with the stability of the spine once the fusion mass is solid.

9. *Will having children cause my curvature to increase with or without surgery for scoliosis?*

   ANSWER: Retrospective studies of patients previously untreated and treated for idiopathic scoliosis have been carried out in an attempt to identify factors which are of prognostic significance in curve progression. No deleterious affects of pregnancy can be demonstrated other than as pregnancy relates in terms of time with normal degenerative changes of aging. In essence then, the long held and erroneous conclusion that patients with scoliosis should not have children has been effectively disspelled.

10. *Is it necessary for every adult with a severe curvature to have surgery?*

    ANSWER: This depends on what is meant by a severe curvature. A curvature which is of significant magnitude, that is to say in excess of 55 or 60° which is clearly progressing in adult life, or which is giving rise to significant symptoms, that is, pain and/or breathing difficulties, certainly should be treated surgically, However, in those instances where there is neither curve progression nor problems which can be directly attributed to the curvature, there is no absolute indication for surgery.

11. *What are some of the problems in leaving scoliosis untreated?*

    ANSWER: This question has adequately been covered in the body of the chapter dealing with the natural history of untreated scoliosis. Experience in untreated patients would suggest that those who have curves of a magnitude in excess of 50 or 60° at skeletal maturity may encounter difficulties with back pain and/or pulmonary compromise depending upon where the curvature is within the spine.

12. *Does every curvature over 20° progress in adulthood?*

    ANSWER: Curves of over 50° frequently progress in adulthood. Those of less than 30° rarely progress in adulthood and in the group between, the experience has been rather mixed, depending to some degree upon the length of the curve, flexibility of the curve at skeletal maturity and rotational elements within the curve itself.

13. *How often should you see your doctor when you have scoliosis as an adult?*

    ANSWER: The reasons for follow-up of scoliosis in adults are: 1. The importance of knowing precisely what happens to that individual; 2. The need to be absolutely certain that the way that scoliosis is presently treated is indeed the optimal method. In general, it is sufficient to follow curves at intervals of approximately five years once a general trend toward either progression or non progression has been established in an adult patient.

14. *Is there anything one can do to prevent problems with scoliosis in adulthood other than surgery?*

    ANSWER: There is no question that programs aimed at general back care, specifically those including exercises to maintain trunk support musculature, do indeed benefit all persons with or without scoliosis. Keeping physically fit does benefit those with scoliosis with or without surgery in terms of minimizing back pain. It is not a solution however for a progressing curve or for serious back pain once it develops. Steps to minimize pulmonary compromise with such measures as avoidance of smoking and exercises for breathing are also of advantage.

PART II
Interviews

To protect the privacy of the people interviewed the names have been changed.

CHAPTER 1

Stand up Straight!

Natalie, Katherine, Caroline and Marlene had surgery both as children and as adults. They clearly point out that physical trauma in childhood such as having to prepare for major surgery, dealing with braces and body casts and then living with a deformity, plays a significant role in their personality development. All four are from middle-class socio-economic backgrounds, had a variety of occupations, most sedentary, yet related comfortably about their feelings regarding scoliosis treatment.

All four women decided to have a second surgery due to pain, fatigue, cosmetic deformity or shortness of breath. After the second surgery their optimism about the future grew. Marlene and Katherine were single and more concerned about their physical appearance than Caroline and Natalie who were married and had children. Caroline wanted more children and opted for a second surgery before another pregnancy to prevent her curvature from getting worse. Common to all these interviews was that in general friends and relations did not understand the emotional impact scoliosis had on their lives.

NATALIE

Born: 1938

"I am angry! I was never out of the care of an orthopedic man for more than five years since I was 14. I've had two extensive fusions and am now fused from T3 through L4 and I am still deformed."

Natalie, born in 1938, is married and the mother of two daughters. Her scoliosis was detected in 1953 at the age of 14. Canadian born, Natalie is presently a school counselor.

"I am angry! I was never out of the care of an orthopedic man for more than five years since I was 14. I've had two extensive fusions and am now fused from T3 through L4 and I am still deformed. I suffered needless years of pain. Ignorance or lack of knowledge has done me in. The first physician I saw in 1953 bristled when he discovered my mother refused to brace me. I left his care in 1964 with the then knowledge that scoliosis didn't progress after physical maturation."

In the fall of 1951 when Natalie was 13 years old, her mother decided to have her scoliosis checked by an orthopedic surgeon. Her scoliosis was detected when she was in ballet class. "I had a Russian ballet mistress who decided that everyone would have to do acrobatics to limber up. I loved ballet and had earned the position of first ballerina. My mother didn't want me to fall behind being number one because the school was going to compile a composite of who did well in acrobatics and ballet. So, I was enrolled in this acrobatic class. It became apparent, quickly, that my back was rigid and that I couldn't bend forward properly. The ballet mistress, who was from the old school of dance, literally *stepped on my back*. I had to do back bends. It turned out that nothing gave in terms of doing back bends except the living room furniture. One day, after practicing for three months to get myself to bend over, I managed to do it. There was this enormous *crack* at the spine. My mother happened to be close by and said, 'Nothing that makes that much noise, could possibly be good for you.' She continued, 'That's it, I don't care whether you are going to be last in the line of ballerinas, that's it!' I said, 'Whewwwwwwsh, thank *God*!' So I crawled up off the floor.

That Christmas my mother decided to make me a vest and skirt. She was an accurate measurer. Things were made from a blueprint. While she measured me, she wanted me to stand in front of her. It was then that she noticed about one-half inch worth of difference in the vest. All the while, she kept saying, 'Stand up straight.' Several weeks later she measured me again and found about an inch difference. She had hit the peak and things were changing fast. My mother, vaguely aware of scoliosis from her training as an anesthetist, then took me to a large medical center for consultation. There, I was referred to a specialist who recommended exercise. My mother was the kind of person, who once making a commitment, always followed through. So, even if she did not particularly like what the doctor said, she followed through. The doctor suggested having me lie on my elbow on my side. Well, two things interfered with that when I tried it. One was that I was in an honors program at school and couldn't spend three hours a night lying on my side doing nothing and finish the program. However, I wasn't bright enough to tell her that! The second problem was that lying like that on my side made me nauseous. Although it really bothered her to hear me complain, she thought, maybe I wasn't giving it 100 per cent. Meanwhile, everytime I would lay on my left side, I would gag. After about a year of continued monthly visits to the doctor, my mother could visually see things worsening.

Somewhere along the way, another specialist was recommended to us. After seeing him, it was decided at the age of 15½ years, that I needed surgery. My first surgery was in 1954 and was an awful psychological experience. I was bedridden for six months. My mother believed in the inside soul. It didn't matter whether I was straight or not, I was not given permission to feel sorry for myself because of the way I looked. Absolutely not! When I had my first surgery, I could have used some counseling just from the point of view of having a real hard task mistress for a mother. It would have been nice to hear, 'It's OK if you don't do it quite as well as *Pollyanna* did it.'

After my surgery, my mother insisted I wear size 12 tops even though I was always on the thin side. I went around for years, through my college and an advertising career, with clothes that just draped over me. I have always found it hard to find clothes that disguised the scoliosis. Until I was 37 years old, I worried about the way I looked in clothes. Then, somehow after that, I decided that if I could be reincarnated, I would want to come back wearing jersey tops! The inconsistency of that just hit me and I thought, this is ridiculous, I'm only trudging through this way once, and I am going to wear what I want!

Upon being told by the orthopedic surgeon who performed my surgery that by the age of 60 I would develop arthritis, I decided that I shouldn't foist any of these problems on anyone else. So, if I'm going to become sick at 60, then I have no business upsetting some poor man's life when one comes along. During my dating years, that's the way I looked at life. I looked around to see if I could find someone who wasn't terribly athletic, since my only athletic interests were swimming and horseback riding.

When I met my husband, Mark, I was nearly 30. He, too, had a physical problem. I felt that was wonderful. He was just what I needed, someone who wasn't totally and extremely healthy. He didn't feel it was fair for him to marry because he didn't know the full extent of his problem at that time. Although we picked each other for the reasons that we did, we had no idea that we had such diametrically opposed methods of dealing with it . . . (laughter). In fact, after 13 years Mark finally commented, 'I think we've finally made it.' At first, I think he was happy with my having scoliosis. As he watched it progress, however, he got embarrassed and didn't know how to approach the subject. About two years ago Mark said to me, 'I was always afraid people wouldn't give you a chance, especially on a job interview.' As a result of that comment, I knew it meant a lot to him.

When Mark measured me, he said that I was 5'5" tall. I said that according to my driver's license, I was 5'6½" tall, which is what I was following my surgery at age sixteen. He insisted that I measured 5'5" and that I should do something about it. But, I remarked, 'What is there to do?' Surgeons that I have seen in the past told me that there is nothing left to do. I was in pain, but not severe pain. I suppose if someone convinced me that I was going to die if I didn't have surgery, I would consider it, otherwise, my experiences from my first surgery left me too traumatized.

That summer, I started my education program at the university in guidance and counseling. I signed up for courses planning to complete my degree. In the middle of July, I called to make an appointment with an orthopedic surgeon to check on my back. In the meantime, Mark continued to measure me. Like my mother, Mark was an accurate measurer. This time he found me to be 5'4½". That was another half-inch off from the last time.

The orthopedic surgeon that examined me felt all that was needed at this time was monitoring. He indicated that surgery was possible, but he first wanted to review past X-rays and compare them with longitudinal X-rays in order to make a decision. I had X-rays taken in 1967 and again in 1971 between pregnancies. After all information was reviewed, the doctor gave me a call. That call came at the end of the summer. A 15 degree difference was noted.

In February of 1979, I cheerfully went back to his office expecting to hear that nothing had changed. With this X-ray, the curve had progressed another 5 degrees. The doctor told me to consider surgery and not to put it off. I wasn't even promised relief from pain, just that it would stop the progression of the curve. I had a big decision to make. With a husband who had meningitis and needed to be transfused and two small children at home ages six and eight, this wouldn't be easy.

My co-workers were telling me, 'Why go through more surgery when you do so well without it? After all, You never know what could happen to you!' I called my doctor and said, 'I'm getting cold feet.' He said something like, 'I'll be waiting.' The thought of him waiting every summer with scapel in hand didn't appeal to me at all. I quickly changed my mind and called back saying, 'I'm coming, I'm coming.' Surgery was scheduled for that May.

The day after checking into the hospital, I was given a general anesthetic and had halo traction inserted into my skull. I also gave my own blood prior to the surgery date. In this spinal fusion, I had a Harrington Rod inserted. After surgery, I was turned on a Stryker Frame. I was feeling some pain, but had no idea what it was. X-rays were taken and I waited anxiously to be put into my first plaster cast. The next morning, I knew something was wrong. At ten o'clock my surgeon came in to tell me he had seen the X-rays and my rod had come loose from the fusion. I felt anger, despair, and depression quickly. The doctor asked if I wanted to have the rod reattached. I answered, no, that I didn't think that I was ready for that, emotionally or physically. I had the cast put on and was released from the hospital on the next Wednesday.

It was now July, and I had the rod taken out with a local anesthetic in the out-patient clinic. After my surgery in 1979, the continuing curvature was halted. There was some cosmetic improvement. After surgery, my doctor asked me if I was still in pain. I said, 'No.' I, truthfully, didn't realize I was in pain before, because I didn't know what the absence of pain felt like. What I did discover was that prior to surgery, I was in pain all the time. Pain, to me, was always divided into two categories, 1) that which I could put up with and 2) that which I could not. When the facet joints were removed for the bone graph, arthritic joints were also removed. Quite a bit of arthritis was responsible for the pain. After the whole back stopped hurting, I could tell that, indeed, I felt different. I have stopped hurting. I have a lot more energy. I can confidently say this now, because when my children were young, I would bend over at least four times a day to pick up toys, but once again I was taught not to complain. I suffer in silence.

At my last visit with my doctor, I dismissed myself. The receptionist stopped me at the door. 'When shall we see you next, Natalie?' I said, 'Next? There isn't going to be a next time!' The doctor overheard the conversation and came out to the reception area with arms folded and a smile on his face. . . . 'I understand,' he said, 'You think you're finished!' "

KATHERINE

Born: 1942

"I guess I would like to have a nice straight back. Scoliosis has been a part of my life for so long that I wouldn't know myself any differently than I am now."

Katherine was born in 1942. She was the youngest of five children: three boys and two girls. Her oldest brother died a year before her first spinal fusion in 1955; he was 23. Her scoliosis was detected at the age of 11. It was her oldest brother who had convinced her mother that she should have surgery. No other treatment was recommended. Following surgery, Katherine wore a cast for a year followed by another year in a brace. In 1974 Katherine had her second spinal fusion.

"As a child, I was very pampered and very much the baby. When I look back at my surgery in 1955, I feel that I was so very passive about it. It was almost like it was an adult problem—not mine. It *was* my parent's problem and I was just the person to whom this was all being done. I remember being afraid in the hospital. I also remember being frustrated and wanting to sit up and my Dad telling me to lie flat. I also remember being able to roll over onto my stomach to feed myself. My cast came just below my neck down to my hips.

The other day I was watching a television program about children going into the hospital for surgery. Things like what to expect when one goes into the hospital and what things will be like during the surgery were explained. That seems so important. When I think back to my surgery, I say, 'Geez, I went in for this big, hairy thing, and no one said a word to me about what was going to happen.'

I feel so much of my thinking is influenced because of my religious background. Every little experience helps make me what I am. I have a hard time, sometimes, separating my feelings about scoliosis from my faith. It is all so intertwined. There is the idea that the *Lord* loves you even more if He gives you a cross to bear. But, that gets a little corny because I don't think that's the case. I do think that people who have a physical problem have to believe that they are viewed as special by the *Lord*.

Yet, on the other hand, I feel kind of proud that I have this *big thing* to deal with. I do not know, to this day, whether or not I use my scoliosis as a cop out. I know I do, sometimes, emotionally. When all my friends were getting married at age 21 or 22 and I was standing up for them, it never occurred to me as to why I wasn't in this boat. Why wasn't someone there waiting for me? It just seemed real normal for it to be happening to everyone else, but me!

I am still very nervous about my back and how it looks to men. I don't feel that I have a pretty body. I know women who are obese, yet they whip out and go to bed with many guys and don't give it a second thought. But, I wonder, how can they do it when it's not even a man they love or who loves them. I will never be completely comfortable undressed in front of anyone—men or women. I guess it is important to try not to be so terribly sensitive. It's like a death, when people say the wrong things.

I think the worst thing about scoliosis is that it happens at the period of time in one's young life when it is difficult to deal with. If one got scoliosis at age 35, there would be more experiences and resources to deal with it better. It's a strange kind of thing. I think it's more difficult because people look at you and say, 'Well, it's not that bad—big deal!' Yet, it is something that has to be taken care of. We do need other people's help and support even if we are soon up and about.

Properly fitting clothing is very important for a person with scoliosis. I won't wear anything real clingy. If I am wearing a bathing suit, I make sure I am always covered, especially if I'm around people I don't know very well. Personally, I feel that if a person with scoliosis doesn't dress well that they feel that they look so awful, anyway.

I guess I would like to have a nice straight back. Scoliosis has been a part of my life for so long that I wouldn't know myself any differently than I am now. The longer I live, the more convinced I am that the pain and suffering that people endure give them strength and empathy for others. I really like myself. I like the kind of person I am striving to be. All this stuff about being youth oriented and being pretty isn't important. What is important is good feelings about yourself, a loving family and good, loyal friends.

I am really so grateful to my parents for taking care of my back. We didn't have a lot of money, yet they still found the best doctor. I would have resented them had they not taken care of this. Based on my personal experience, I wouldn't hesitate to encourage *anyone,* child or adult, to have the surgery if that was what was recommended by their surgeon.

I decided to have my back checked again when I began having pain, experiencing fatigue and shortness of breath about 1973. Of course, I was apprehensive, knowing what I had been through years ago, but I was assured that medicine had made great strides in the field of scoliosis, since my first spinal fusion in 1955. The degree of my curve was increasing and was measured at 90 degrees. I was afraid that I would be told that nothing could be done.

This time, I went out-of-state for an opinion. I was told by the surgeon that I could have a second surgery using halo-femoral traction to allow maximum correction for my rigid curve. There would be two surgeries: one to break down the first fusion and insert the halo-femoral traction, and the second to do the spinal fusion. The correction, I was told, would be to about 56 degrees. I decided to have it done as soon as possible. It was probably easier for me to make the decision because I was single.

After my second surgery, I felt like I was reborn. Now, I have a fairly good self-image. It's not real great, but fairly good. Since my surgery in 1974, I acquired a new job. I am presently in sales where I make a lot of cold calls. This entails getting in and out of my car constantly, doing a lot of driving, carrying a briefcase, and being on my feet a good deal of the day. I do this, now, absolutely free of pain and tiredness, something that would not have been possible before my second surgery.

I feel that being touched with a serious problem like scoliosis, one becomes more sensitive to the needs of others. I was determined to make scoliosis a positive experience for me. The encouragement and support I received, and the love shown to me during that very difficult period, will *never* be forgotten and *never* taken for granted. It's an awfully good feeling to know that something tough has been asked of you, and you made it through!"

CAROLINE

Born: 1951

"Whenever I am in a situation where I haven't seen people in a long time, I just cringe when they approach me with a hug. Most people do not understand the hangups that scoliosis patients have about their appearance."

Caroline was born in 1951. Her scoliosis was detected at age eleven, she had surgery at age 12 and again at 31. Presently, Caroline is a housewife and mother of three children. The doctor who treated Caroline as a child made no mention as to the possibility that her curvature might progress as an adult and further surgery would be needed. Because she wanted to have more children, Caroline considered surgery before her third pregnancy to stop the progression of her increasing scoliosis. Caroline is one of four children in her family: two boys and two girls. She and her sister have scoliosis. Caroline noticed the scoliosis on her sister a couple of years after her own spinal fusion as a child. Although they both knew it was apparent, they kept it quiet from their parents because Caroline's sister didn't want them to have to go through the trauma of surgery a second time.

"I had my spinal fusion when I was 12 years old. Prior to my surgery I did exercises to improve my curve. But, my curve was too large for exercise alone to make a difference. One doctor suggested wearing a Milwaukee Brace, but the doctor we ended up seeing insisted on operating. I cannot remember being in any pain, just discomfort wearing a body cast for six months. In fact, I don't even remember being self-conscious about my back through high school. I wore bathing suits. It was just recently that I have become more self-conscious about the progressing hump in the lumbar area.

Recently, at a party, a friend came over to me and put his arm around my waist resting his arm on the hump. 'Good *Lord*,' he said, 'what is that?' I explained to him that I had scoliosis. Whenever I am in a situation where I haven't seen people in a long time, I just cringe when they approach me with a hug. Most people do not understand the hangups that scoliosis patients have about appearance. I try not to accentuate any bad part of me, so basically, people are not aware of my scoliosis upon first seeing me. I find that I am very self-conscious now about my appearance. The Scoliosis Association of Michigan has played an important role in my life. Finally, I have found a place where my work will help others as well as myself.

I really didn't experience any problems with my pregnancies. In fact, I really felt my best. It wasn't until I went into labor that I began to experience lower back pain. But, from what I hear talking with other women going through natural childbirth, that is a common problem, scoliosis or not. The doctors felt that if I was going to experience any pain, it would be from the additional weight on my spine. On May 20, 1981, I delivered a 9 lb. 3 oz. baby girl, naturally. I also have a two year old.

The last time that I had X-rays was about three or four years ago. There was no apparent change in the thoracic curve, but the lumbar curve showed some progression. I do plan to have this checked out. At that time, I thought about not having children. I didn't want to pass scoliosis on to them. But, Bill, my husband, changed my mind. He felt that scoliosis was not a good enough reason for not having children. Since I made it through my life just fine, there was no reason to deny us the pleasure of having children just on the *chance* that they may get scoliosis. My life has changed a lot in the past five years. I enjoy being at home, taking care of my children, and having something to work for by helping others."

(*After the delivery of Caroline's second child, she made an appointment with an orthopedic surgeon. She was scheduled for surgery that spring.*) "My surgery as an adult was quite scary, especially since my children were ages one and three. Everyone helped, however. Friends and family included. My three year old became my private nurse and we all grew much closer. My husband was my tower of strength. Positive thinking got us through the whole ordeal. If one can discount the fact that surgery is a temporary condition in comparison to the rest of one's life, it becomes worth it. Life is just too short to pass up a chance to change a situation—something one shouldn't leave behind."

MARLENE

Born: 1943

"A person with scoliosis needs a tough hide, a high self-esteem, and a good sense of humor to survive in our society."

Marlene was born in 1943, has had two spinal fusions—one in 1955 and the other in 1981. Her scoliosis was detected at the age of 9 as a result of polio. Marlene's mother died at the age of 54. She had severe scoliosis due to polio. Marlene is single. She has one brother who does not have scoliosis.

"I had my first surgery at 12. At the time my little brother was 6 years old. I was brought home from the hospital in an ambulance and was wearing a body cast that extended from my neck down one leg. When I was brought into the house on a stretcher, I asked to see my brother. My parents looked all over for him and found him in the yard crying. When he finally came inside, I heard him saying, 'Marlene can't walk. She's never going to walk.' I yelled out to him, 'I'm OK, I'm OK!' That night, he brought his pillow and blankets and camped out on the floor next to my bed and went to sleep. In the fall when he was supposed to start school, I was still bedridden. He refused to leave me to go to school.

My mother took care of me at home from August to the following January. Then I was moved to a convalescent home because I needed a lot of care and was to lie flat on my back. It was difficult to maintain my social life laid up in bed for as long as I was. I didn't make many friends during my scoliosis surgery and recuperation period to follow. I had occupational therapy in the hospital. I hated it with a passion. I was in pain while being asked to twist with a cast on. I wouldn't eat the food in the hospital, either. The dietician came up to see me to make some special arrangements for food. I was in the hospital from May to August.

I graduated from college in 1972 and have changed professions twice since. I think having scoliosis has made me demand more from myself. I'm not happy just being mediocre. I want the kind of job that will make me happy as a career person. I feel just as normal as anyone else, except when it comes to the job market. I feel that's where I am discriminated against the most due to scoliosis. Secondly, I feel I cannot attract the kind of guys that I like because I can't do what they expect me to do. I get too pooped out! I just cannot go dancing all night to the wee hours.

The only thing that has kept me going through all of this is my intelligence. I've always rationalized the whole thing. If something is bad now, I always think, that's now! I always look at my life in terms of a whole, I don't look at one little aspect. I see my life as going on and on like months, years, etc.

The deformity that accompanies scoliosis has affected me both professionally and socially. I have applied for many executive secretarial positions only to be turned down after the interview. They are most impressed with my resume but once they meet me, my qualifications seem to dwindle before their eyes. I did become an executive secretary, but one victory doesn't erase all those rejections. Once I was in line for secretary to the President of the company, but was refused consideration without reason even though I had been his secretary for four months. I sat and watched the parade of candidates pass my desk and enter his office. Socially, I feel my deformity frightens many men off before I can even say "hello." I am, unfortunately, pursued by men who only want 'a good time.' Many men seem to think a woman with a deformity has little if any morality, and that she should be grateful for any attention given to her. One man told me he went out with me for curiosity. Scoliosis is a real handicap when you are looking for a husband.

There is little wonder, then, that psychological problems arise. A person with scoliosis needs a tough hide, a high self-esteem, and a good sense of humor to survive in our society. And, where does one go for help? A doctor told me a year ago, that he never intended for me to work when he released me at the age of 18. How did he expect me to earn a living? A psychologist told me to quit my job and go back to college to get my master's degree. What did he expect me to live on in the meantime? It's a real world out there—and a changing one.

I went back to the doctor to check on my back when severe pain set in. I am always so careful with my health. I guess I was most worried about developing respiratory problems. If I would get a cold, I would stay home until it was all gone. I won't push myself. But the back pain I was now experiencing made me fight harder. My boss would tell me to go home. By the time I gave in, surgery was the only answer.

My father came to stay with me during my second surgery in August of 1981. My curve had progressed to 137 degrees. When I had my first surgery in 1955, my curve was measured at 90 degrees. With this surgery, I had to wear halo-traction with my cast before and after surgery. I decided to continue my life as best I could. I had to go on disability with the promise I could get a position with the same company when I was ready to come back to work. My doctor said I would be able to do most anything when the cast came off.

To me all that has happened in my life seems to be the norm—having polio, being in a convalescent home, hospitals, etc. If nothing happens, bad or good, one would be bored. Although I expect to still have some discomfort following this surgery, I am optimistic. I think, now, I will take life easy, perhaps concentrate more on my writing poetry and doing gourmet cooking."

CHAPTER **2**

It Could Be Worse!
Living with Pain

The eleven adults interviewed in this chapter have had a variety of treatments for scoliosis but none have had surgery. Their ages range from the early thirties to early eighties. These individuals clearly point out that the physical trauma experienced in their early childhood development played a significant role in their personality development.

Miles, who was born in 1902, and Cora, born in 1906, both felt that as the years went by, their curvatures became more obvious. Neither felt that having scoliosis prevented them from being all that they hoped to become. Both are active and productive people leading interesting and active lives. Miles is presently a real estate agent and Cora a retired bookkeeper and secretary to the Dean of a University.

Freida, born in 1921, Imogene, born in 1923, Frank, born in 1928, Eli, born in 1931, and Marge, born in 1938, were very sensitive about their cosmetic appearance. They all felt that not only was their deformity more pronounced as years went by, but also more difficult to conceal. All experienced reduced stamina, shortness of breath, and limitations with regard to physical activity.

Shirley, born 1952, Cassie, born 1956, and Bonnie, born 1959, had a great deal more repressed anger. They all believed there was an end to their treatment and were disappointed to find that their curvatures had progressed as adults. They all are in the stage of talking to others, seeking out information, and getting more opinions. All are apprehensive about surgery, yet they are not satisfied with the status quo.

MILES

Born: 1902

"I still get excellent reports of good health from physical examinations. My first night in a hospital came about from an auto accident at age 79."

Miles was born in 1902 and grew up on a farm. He was about 12 years old when scoliosis was detected. He recalls walking down a dirt road to get to the town store when he came upon a friend of his walking behind him. He called out to him saying, "Hey there fellow, you are carrying one shoulder higher than the other." Another of his recollections was walking home from the fields with his hands crossed, one over the other. His grandfather asked him if he had a sore back. Apparently it had become noticeable, but no further mention was made. Miles comments that out of his fifty cousins, no one else has scoliosis. In fact, he has three grown children and none have scoliosis.

"I did see a doctor about the problem when I was about 17 years old," Miles remarked. "He ordered a brace which arrived parcel post and cost, then, about thirty-five dollars. I was working in the mail room of the post office at the time it arrived. My boss remarked that I was well built for football and didn't understand my need for the brace. He was sincere, but quite surprised when I explained that I needed the brace for a back problem. The brace in the package contained two printed sheets of highly technical instructions for exercises to strengthen each of several muscles. I could not understand the vocabulary. The doctor I was seeing, the high school coach, and the YMCA coach could not help me decipher the information either. I did try to wear the brace for about 3 months, but with no success.

From the age of 25 to 35 years, I had pains in my right leg. However, in recent years the pain subsided. I do have some knee and muscle problems, but this may be due to my age rather than scoliosis.

Scoliosis did not prevent me from obtaining a career choice; presently I am a realtor, property manager and retired headmaster. Scoliosis did keep me out of state civil service, however. It does occasionally slow me down a bit, but I still manage a minimum of eight hours weekly in club and lodge meetings.

I really didn't think much about scoliosis because I have always been very busy. I did feel it became more obvious to others after age 50, but I could still disguise it in tailored suits. Although I have always considered myself rather average in looks, at age 18 or so, I did feel that I was less attractive due to scoliosis.

I still get excellent reports of good health from physical examinations. My first night in a hospital came about from an auto accident at age seventy nine."

CORA

Born: 1906

"One thing to be thankful for today, when looking back at my past, is that scoliosis is being checked early."

Cora was born in 1906, a premie with congenital scoliosis. She has four children and none have scoliosis. One of her daughters has a very small degree of curvature. She does have one granddaughter with scoliosis that has been treated with a brace.

"One thing to be thankful for today, when looking back at my past, is that scoliosis is being checked early. Of course, we had physical exams while in school, and my parents never let a day go by without reminding me to 'stand up straight.' At first my Dad thought I was careless and a bit sloppy about my posture. When I got bad reports at school regarding my physical, I blamed myself, but, couldn't correct it. I wore braces, one after another. We lived in California and my dad took me to every specialist available. My mother had a dressmaker make all my clothes. They were always adjusted to the one side that was shorter than the other.

Scoliosis really hasn't changed my life. I still earned my degree, I have a Master's Degree in Business Education. I have been a bookkeeper and also worked at a university as the secretary to the Dean of the Music School.

A while back I was having severe back problems and pain. The doctor tried putting me in a brace. But, I absolutely could not wear it. It was too high. I could walk with it on, but could not sit. If I had continued to wear that brace, I wouldn't have been able to get around at all. At this point, I am not going to take the chance of even cutting a month out of my life to try something that would set me back. My greatest fear is that I will not be able to move about on my own. My back is getting worse and the pain more intense. However, I feel that determination, good attitude, good family support is what it takes to maintain a good and positive self-image."

FREIDA

Born: 1921

"The moment I get bitter about having scoliosis and the problems associated with it, I just stop and count my blessings."

Born in Munich, Germany in 1921, Freida was 14 years old when her family doctor discovered scoliosis and referred her to an orthopedic clinic. The first thing that was done was to put her in a cast from under her arms to her hips for six weeks.

Freida comments: "I was on an exercise program during that time. After six weeks, the cast was removed. Then I had another cast made that was removable and molded to my body. On the side where I had the hump, pressure was applied, pushing it in. After five years, there was no improvement. I continued with an extensive exercise program of stretching and swimming. I began to play tennis, but gave it up because I was warned that one-sided exercises built up muscles on one side. Then the war came in Germany, many doctors were called to the military. That was it for treatment.

I was the eldest of three girls in my family. We were all very close. My sisters wouldn't let me do any work at home. They were very protective. One day, as I bent over to lift a bucket, my sister shouted for my mother, 'Look, come look at what Freida has on her back.' Apparently, the hump was very noticeable. A year before that incident, I came down with diphtheria and then had an allergic reaction to the serum. I was very, very ill. Afterward, I had a very thorough physical and at that time, even my family doctor saw nothing, he just listened to my lungs.

If I didn't have scoliosis or any noticeable deformity, it would have changed my life, I'm sure. I probably would have stayed in my nursing profession which I gave up because of the strain on my back. I also had a friend who was a tennis pro. We started seeing a lot of each other and fell in love. While swimming one day, he told me that since he was a sports pro he had to have a wife who first could play tennis with him, and secondly a wife who had a good figure. I was crushed. But, looking back, that was probably the best thing that could have happened. For, with those values, who knows how long that marriage would have lasted. Yes, my life would have been very different.

The most negative effect scoliosis has had on me is when it comes to selecting clothes. I learned to sew and make my own clothes and adjustments. I am not real comfortable in a bathing suit, but I wear one anyway because I love to swim. When I am traveling and have to swim in the hotel pool, I take my robe with me, take it off and leave it right next to the poolside. Then, I go in the water and swim. When I come out, I take my towel, my robe and put it on and go directly to a chair. I am sure that there are people with other kinds of shapes—both good and bad, that make people turn around and stare. But, I am sure that I am more sensitive and conscious of it than others are.

I am a very ambitious person always trying harder to achieve goals. I used to be a secretary in the American Consulate in Germany. When I came to America I got a job as a secretary in a large firm. I had good command of English and other foreign languages. That was an advantage.

I really didn't have any pain with scoliosis until I was about 30. I started having severe pain in my left ribs. The doctor prescribed a lumbosacral back brace. I wore it conscientiously for a year because it really helped.

I try to stay as healthy as I can by staying in shape, looking my best, and looking as young as I can for as long as I can. The moment I get bitter about having scoliosis and the problems associated with it, I just stop and count my blessings. I have the good fortune to weigh the good things in life that have happened—good parents, good sisters, good friends, a loving husband, and the financial security to be able to enjoy life to its fullest. These far outweigh the bad with scoliosis. Everyone has something that troubles them and we all feel sorry for ourselves once in a while. I stop and look at the good and say, I deserve those things too!"

MARTHA

Born: 1924

"I think in this country, especially, we are visually oriented from infancy. I don't imagine that a lot of people are willing to admit it, but they have preconceived notions of what normal men and women, boys and girls should look like. When people deviate from that too much, there is trouble."

Martha was born in 1924 and has idiopathic scoliosis. She has two sons. Neither one has scoliosis. Martha recalls that prior to the polio vaccine, her sister was bedridden with a virus. Her family doctor felt that she and her sister may have had a mild case of polio.

"Most of the time my low back is aching. This usually occurs after I've done some walking or have been on my feet for any length of time. I used to let out some of my pain in music. I played the violin and piano. My husband seems to feel that my playing the violin had a lot to do with the pain.

Clothes just recently have become a problem. I've always had to have my clothes altered, but I've worn them loosely even before scoliosis became obvious. I think in this country, especially, we are visually oriented from infancy. I don't imagine that a lot of people are willing to admit it, but they have preconceived notions of what normal men and women, boys and girls should look like. When people deviate from that too much, there is trouble.

I say scoliosis doesn't bother me. Yet, I am very conscious when I meet someone I haven't seen in a long time, and they give me a big hug or run their hand down my back. In fact, even when my husband does that, I wonder if it puts him off. He has never said much about it, but I still wonder.

I think it would be really great if I could learn to tolerate the pain without any medication. I have increasing trouble with my housework. The pain becomes very sharp in my back. I try to exercise about a half hour each morning with body toning and developing back muscles. When the pain increases, I stop and rest. Physical appearance does not concern me as much as pain. I guess I just have to build up a tolerance for this and accept the fact that this is just the way things will be!"

FRANK

Born: 1928

"What bothered me all my life was the appearance of my back. There was nothing I could do to hide it. I definitely considered it a cross to bear all my life."

Frank was born in 1928. He is one of ten children. His scoliosis was detected at the age of eight by a nun in the parochial school he attended. Other than observation, there has been no treatment.

"I blame what I am on the misfortune of having scoliosis. What else can I blame it on? I can't blame my mother and father because they weren't educated enough to rush their child to a doctor immediately like modern day parents do. I really believe that my parents felt this was an act of *God* and nothing could be done.

I used to be an altar boy. After services, the nun would say, 'Come here, let me see you.' She would be looking at my shoulders from the back. I also remember my dad checking shoulder levels, or whatever he noticed. I don't believe that the nun or my dad suspected scoliosis. I don't think they knew what the word meant.

When I was in the eighth grade, scoliosis became more obvious and severe. My mother took me to a hospital clinic where I had X-rays taken. The only treatment prescribed was exercise. But, after doing them for a couple of months to no avail, I stopped. The problem had progressed too far at that time for exercise alone to do any good.

I am very self-conscious about my scoliosis. My legs appear to be a lot longer in proportion to the rest of my body. I sometimes wear my shirt outside of my belt to conceal my short-waisted torso. What really bothered me all my life is the appearance of my back. There was nothing I could do to hide it. Scoliosis has had a definite effect on me. In my estimation it made me introverted and an outcast. I definitely considered it a cross to bear all my life. No question about it. It affected my life from my teenage years on when it became noticeable to me. I never thought I was good looking. Years ago I was quite thin in addition to having scoliosis. I looked sickly and pale. I try to be objective about it, but looking back at pictures, I look like I had some dreadful disease.

I've had a very unhappy life due to scoliosis. I am and always was extremely self-conscious about my appearance. I am not married because I'm sure that women considered me unattractive. Scoliosis has presented some limitations, not physical though. It has kept me from going on further and seeking promotions and so forth. There is not much that I can't do physically like lifting or manual labor. I've done quite a bit of machine shop work, woodworking, things like that. I've indicated that I don't have the strength and I have limited lung capacity. So I tire easily and have a faster heart rate.

When I was 21, I went to a hospital to have my back checked again. At that time, I was told that there was really nothing more that could be done. That was the end of that. Up until I attended a Scoliosis Association of Michigan meeting one winter, I wasn't aware that anything could be done. I didn't even know that a curve could be measured.

My lifetime goals have changed somewhat. I don't have the strong urge to marry as I did 20 years ago. I would get married now, if I found a compatible woman, but I don't go seeking out that person. Presently, I am looking forward to retiring from my teaching job and taking life easy."

ELI

Born: 1931

"During a disagreement my wife said to me, 'That hump really turns me off and I can't stand that.' She was angry and I guess to my dying day, I will never know how much is her true feelings or just below the belt to hurt."

Eli was born in 1931. He is married and has three children. When he was 14 years old his mother took him to an orthopedic surgeon who prescribed a corset-like garment which eventually broke, proved worthless, and was discarded. The doctor he is presently seeing for his scoliosis indicated that it could have an effect on his heart and lungs if it continues to increase. Eli feels that the pain he is experiencing now is chronic. "I get up in the morning with it and I go to bed with it at night. I take aspirin when the pain gets real bad. I can do things, but I can't last as long or do them as well. It has been getting worse. Lately, I seem more frustrated with the pain. Perhaps it is scoliosis related, but probably more so due to age. One really must take a good look at oneself.

This has been the worst year for me. I guess I am more sensitive about my scoliosis. It has become more noticeable to me and more painful. I think one of the reasons I am so uncomfortable this year in particular is that I have added 20 pounds to my weight. Comments have been made by the kids in the school where I teach. I believe they are good natured comments, but nonetheless they refer to my *hump back*. A couple of kids in particular have said to me, 'Hey, what's the matter?' I try to be open when I discuss my back and let them know that the curvature is getting worse. They can see that I am in pain. One kid patted me on the back and said, 'How's Ol' man hump back?' Generally, nothing is said.

Husbands and wives sometimes have disagreements—my wife and I are no different. But this one stands out in my mind as a real humdinger! My wife sparked at me, 'That hump really turns me off and I can't stand that.' I know she was angry and I guess to my dying day, I will never know how much was her true feelings or just below the belt to hurt. She and my sons will sometimes say, 'Hey, Dad, you never spend any time with us,' or 'we never see you and we want to do things with you.' When they do see me, I am either running, or dead to the world. These are not my *druthers*, I would much rather spend time with them. But the two jobs I work at provide the things they like to do. I'm afraid that is very frustrating.

I always walk to the synagogue on Saturday. Once in a while a member will pass me by in a car and ask if I'd like a ride because I walk with my hand on my back and my face is filled with pain. I always refuse. The pain is increasing daily. I just have to sit down and rest more frequently these days.

There is no question that I am different and my scoliosis is noticeable. *It ain't no blessing.* Complain and you'll either get drugged up with medication, or face the fact that surgery is the answer. My advice is don't wait until major problems develop, take care of your scoliosis early!"

IMOGENE

Born: 1923

"I love shopping for clothes, but get so disappointed with the way they fit."

Imogene was born in 1923 and is an only child. She is married and has no children. Her scoliosis was discovered when she was 13 years old. It was her mother that took her to an orthopedic surgeon who said there was nothing that could be done for her scoliosis. That was in 1936. It was never discussed any further in her family.

"I don't like having scoliosis. I am not happy about it. As a result I have developed an inferiority complex and am very shy. I don't like to speak in front of people and I don't like people to look at me. I always think that maybe people feel sorry for me because of my deformity.

My mom and dad are divorced. My father liked to run around. He was very good looking and was very disappointed in my looks. I remember an incident at the restaurant when I was 21 years old. He turned to me and said, 'You know, Imogene, you don't look so bad after all.' I felt, at that point, it would have been better if he didn't say anything at all.

Scoliosis has had a negative effect on my self-image. But, I'd probably be critical even if I didn't have scoliosis. I love shopping for clothes, but get so disappointed with the way they fit. This reminds me of a story that happened to me in my early 20's when I was asked to stand up at a girlfriend's wedding. I told her I'd take the same dress that all the other bridesmaids were wearing. One of the bridesmaids told me that the bride's sister felt that I would ruin the wedding party because of my back. As a result they couldn't pick out the dresses that they really wanted. It was too late for me to back out, the dresses were in.

The pain isn't that severe that I can't live with it. There are times when it is more pronounced because I have developed spurs on my spine which cause occasional pressure on nerves making it difficult to walk. When I go to the doctor for a check-up on my back, I always ask, what's going to happen when I get older? My spine is severely curved at 78 degrees right thoracic. I have seen people whose backs look worse than mine, yet their degree of curvature is not as great as mine. I have also noticed that the right side is sticking out more and my left side is going in more. The other day I saw a coat that I just fell in love with. I waited for my husband to see it with me. He remarked that it puckered on the right side. I was heartbroken.

I still do everything I enjoy doing such as gardening, housework, playing cards, traveling, etc. I tire a little more easily, but quite honestly, I don't really have any limitations."

MARGE

Born: 1938

*"I think that I would have more self-confidence if
I didn't have scoliosis, because I wouldn't have to
always be thinking about how I look."*

Marge was born in 1938. She is the mother of four girls all of whom have scoliosis to some degree. Her scoliosis was first noticed at the age of 16.

"Having scoliosis is a pain! I knew my body was crooked when I was about 16 years old and trying on bathing suits. I loved one particular suit and almost bought it when I caught a glimpse of myself from the side in a mirror. No matter how I stood the suit fit me on a slant. I was sick inside, knowing something was seriously wrong with my body. I had no idea it could ever be corrected. I've always been quite aware of my good and bad points and have developed, as a result, a flair for camouflage. I think that I would have more self-confidence if I didn't have scoliosis because I wouldn't have to constantly be thinking about how I look.

When I worked in a fashionable women's apparel shop, maybe 14 or 15 years ago, women would come in with these beautiful bodies and lots of money. One would think that these women had everything, yet they would be so fussy, so critical. 'I don't like the collar like this,' they would say. They'd walk out dissatisfied, cranky, and fussing under their noses. I'd think, 'Lady, do you realize how lucky you are?' One learns to appreciate the good things in life. When I buy an outfit that really fits me well, it really makes my day, my month, sometimes even longer!

I do have limitations because of pain. I can just do so much, walk so far, and lift so much. If I am on my feet an awfully long time, the pain becomes unbearable. I have a lot of pain at the top of the curvature near my neck going down my left shoulder blade. I also get severe migraine headaches. I guess what bothers me the most is that now I am in my prime of life, so to speak, and I never knew that what I suffered with all these years could be corrected. I pray that my scoliosis does not seriously disable me as the years take their toll."

SHIRLEY

Born: 1952

"I feel it is important to look at yourself positively and try to understand what is happening to you. Seek out other people with the similar problem, ask questions, and choose your doctor wisely."

Shirley, born in Canada in 1952, is married with no children. Because of socialized medicine in Canada, the bracing didn't cost her family anything. Shirley had physiotherapy before and after brace treatment to strengthen weak muscles and to learn correct breathing. She also was seen by a social worker who helped her work through the acceptance process of brace wearing. Scoliosis was detected by her mother when Shirley was a young child. She thought it was her posture and wanted her to wear elastics to keep her straight.

"I was always tall for my age. I am now 5'7". In the 9th grade I suddenly had a lot of pain and couldn't carry my books home with me. I'd stop in the middle of the road to sit down. I remember crying all the way home. The dull pain that I had taken for granted, suddenly became real bad and I realized something was wrong. That was the pain that finally led my mother and me to get medical attention.

How your family responds to your scoliosis and to your treatment is going to determine how you turn out. At the end of the 9th grade, I got my brace. At this point, I started feeling real ugly in the brace. The brace had a padded chin rest with uprights on the back of my neck to keep my head from falling forward. The clothes I wore over the brace made me look like a house. My mother found a woman who designed a dress pattern which enabled me to put my clothes over the brace and still allow the bars to come out. Just recently I saw a girl on the bus wearing a Milwaukee Brace. Mine looked nothing like that. I did, however, adjust very quickly to wearing the brace. I had the summer with it before I had to go back to school. I not only was entering the 10th grade, I was entering a new school.

I think the experience of brace wearing helped me grow emotionally. If I had not worn a brace, I probably would have been more shy. This was like an introduction for people to talk to me—make me feel special. Also, scoliosis day in our doctor's office meant bringing a thermos and sandwiches. Everyone with scoliosis came on the same day. It was like a support group. We didn't mind waiting to see the doctor which sometimes meant two to three hours. Everyone would get together to share ideas and stories.

The doctors who treated me thought I may have had a mild case of polio. The area of Canada where I lived had flooding. As a result, many cases of polio were diagnosed.

Although my scoliosis didn't improve much from the 30 degrees at which it was diagnosed, bracing did hold it and keep it from getting worse. I feel it is important to look at yourself positively and try to understand what is happening to you. Seek out other people with similar problems, take the time to ask questions, and choose your doctor wisely. Most importantly, don't be afraid to get a second opinion."

BONNIE

Born: 1959

"When I first found out I had scoliosis, I thought the Lord was punishing me for something."

Bonnie was born in 1959. She is single. Her scoliosis was discovered by accident when she had gone to the doctor for a cold. X-rays were taken. The doctor noticed on the X-rays a problem with her spine and sent her to a specialist.

"I didn't understand anything about scoliosis until I read about it in the paper and attended a Scoliosis Association of Michigan meeting. I went to see an orthopedic surgeon who did suggest surgery. But, at that time I wasn't 21 years old yet and he felt it could be observed for a few years. Right now my curve measures 60 degrees.

I've had problems finding work. My dad works in the post office. I put in an application there, took all the tests and applied in a post office near my home. I was called in to talk with the boss. He said I would be lifting mail bags which weigh approximately 7 pounds each and would be carrying them several feet. After he reviewed my medical report, I received a letter which explained the law suits from people who have bad backs resulting from constant lifting. Every day the jobs had to be rotated, and eventually there could be problems. The bottom line was that they just didn't want to take the risk of hiring me because of my back. I could have fought that because the money was good, but I let the matter drop.

I am very self-conscious about having scoliosis. I've been dating the same guy for about three years now. Every once in a while we talk about my scoliosis because it gets me down. He doesn't find it a problem and tries to get me out of my depressed mood.

When I was working as a waitress, I had to carry a large tray above me. Last December, I started getting really sharp pains on my lower side. It had to be from that lifting. I thought I was really ruining my back, so I quit. Now, I am doing secretarial work in a two-girl office.

When I first found out that I had scoliosis, I thought the *Lord* was punishing me for something. I don't think that way anymore because there are a lot of people with it besides me. I didn't realize that before.

Although I am still undecided about surgery, I do wonder what will happen to me 30 years from now. I really would like to have surgery before I get married, because I just wouldn't want to burden my husband with taking care of me. Anyway, right now I can't afford to take time off from work. I need to feel a little more financially secure."

CASSIE

Born: 1956

"It could be worse . . . It could be worse! Think of all those people who have problems worse than you. That used to make me feel so damned guilty!"

Cassie was born in 1956. She is single. Her scoliosis was detected at the age of nine and was treated with a Milwaukee Brace. Her mother saw signs of scoliosis when Cassie was four and mentioned it to the pediatrician who just kind of dismissed it for the time being. When she was nine he recommended that she be seen by a specialist.

"It could be worse . . . It could be worse! Think of all those people who have problems worse than you. That used to make me feel so *damned guilty!* There is no reason for me to feel guilty about feeling badly. I mean if I were allowed to let out that I am feeling angry or sad—I wouldn't be in it for very long. But, the moment that I would start to say something about it, that I am angry or I don't like being this way, I was told, 'It could be worse.'

When I was a little kid we knew very little about scoliosis. I always felt that I had done something wrong because I couldn't stand up straight. I remember when I heard the doctor discuss with my mother that I was going to be put into a brace, the first thing that I did was bolt up straight in the chair thinking that if I sit like that until my next appointment I'll fix it myself. I was scared to death. I was told that I would be in a Milwaukee Brace for three years or so. When I stopped growing, it would come off, and I would be fine. The doctor mentioned surgery as a way out there, kind of possibility, but nothing to concern myself with now. I did wear the brace. When I got out of it, I thought I was done. I never even thought I'd be thinking about having surgery. . . . I am so pleased that I am able to make the decision about having or not having surgery myself, as an adult. I would rather deal with the problems myself than have to deal with my mother, too, going through the turmoil.

There are four of us in the family. Three girls and one boy. My sisters and brother are all quite a bit older than I. If my parents had stopped with the three—there wouldn't have been any scoliosis. I wore a brace for three years during the most critical time of my growing up years—the time when you get to know boys, get to go to dances, and get involved in activities. I didn't get to do that stuff. I guess I feel sort of *robbed* of a significant adolescent experience. Perhaps, I never caught up.

When I told my sister that I was thinking about going through with surgery, she just played it down. I felt that no one should have to be saddled with this major decision at the age of 23 and no one should have to make such a life-changing decision. It's just not fair. She looked at me and gave me this off-handed answer like 'If it wasn't your back, then it was my eyes.' The response as I understood it was don't make such a big deal out of it.

I really admire parents who let their children express anger. My religious background has trained me to 'offer it up to the *Lord*.' You know, you'll get a spot in heaven. It could be worse! Anger and hostility is less harmful if it is allowed to be expressed. If you can ventilate it, it lessens the feelings and lets them out in the open. But, if it is not allowed, then you learn never to deal with these emotions. It then starts to come out in other ways like depression, bitterness or pseudo-strength. I am in therapy now, and I recommend it highly for scoliosis patients because I feel we all have a lot of buried anger which has to surface.

I feel very much like an adolescent. Many times, I have to force myself to remember that I am an adult just like all these other people I am dealing with. Sometimes I feel like I am the little kid who has been invited to sit and listen, when I am with a group of people. I really feel that I have a three-year deficit. I think it's because scoliosis hits us as an adolescent. It hits us hard. I remember getting out of my brace and feeling that my friends had done things in those years that I wore the brace that I hadn't done. It's almost like a big secret of which I wasn't a part.

I have always had a low opinion of myself. When I was in college, I didn't think that I could handle what I really wanted to do and that was to become a physical therapist. I had trouble with the hard sciences. For the first time in my life, I did *average,* which scared the crap out of me. Since I couldn't handle failure, I went into something that was a little easier, or that I perceived to be easier.

I do feel sort of special, however. I feel real looked at. When I tell people that I have scoliosis, they tell me they would never have noticed or known if I hadn't mentioned it. But, I feel that it is the first thing people do notice.

I would have loved to have been a little bit taller. This is just a projection because I really don't know how a tall person feels. Perhaps it would help me not to feel so much like a *little girl.* I am 5'2" and would just love to be 5'5". As my first doctor told me, I would have been 3 inches taller without scoliosis. Just think, I have an opportunity at the age of 26 to be gangly all over again—like my adolescent years!

I am not in pain. However, I am not sure when I experience something if it is due to scoliosis aches or human being aches. I don't really blame any one thing for being what I am or what I am not. I could point the finger at a lot of things: my rigid upbringing, my place in the family (being the youngest), my father's dying when I was two. I think they all played a real big part in it. But, the important thing is that from here on out, I take responsibility for what I am. I can't express enough the importance of letting feelings air and ventilate. It dilutes them."

CHAPTER **3**

Accentuating the Positive

Body image plays a very important part in the life of any individual. This is especially true when one must live with a deformity such as scoliosis. Sociability and overall self-worth is diminished when one lacks a positive attitude about oneself. This may come about either because of the reactions of the public to the individual or from pre-existing views of one's past body image. To perceive oneself as a sexually attractive individual, one must have developed good feelings of self-worth. That in turn comes from a loving and supportive family relationship.

The six women interviewed in this chapter: Sharon, Brenda, Dorene, Elaine, Sylvia and Marion had surgery as children and have been told they would just have to live with their condition which further contributed to their feelings of isolation. Their past experiences tell them that to complain about one's lot in life serves no purpose because no one will listen. As a result they have developed high thresholds for pain and have selected sedentary types of employment from librarian to social worker.

SHARON

Born: 1943

"I remember when I started dating and going to dances and parties I'd be so self-conscious. When it came time to dance, I'd get tense because that meant my partner would have to put his hand on my body."

Sharon was born in 1943. She is the mother of three boys and one girl none of whom have scoliosis. Her scoliosis was discovered at the age of nine when she started having pain in her hip. She was taken to doctors all over the city trying to determine what was wrong. No one ever mentioned the word scoliosis. Her treatment started off with exercise. Eventually they learned about a doctor at a major medical center who was treating scoliosis. It was there that she had her surgery at the age of 12.

"Scoliosis has been a part of me for so long that I have learned to compensate in social situations. When I talk to people, or when I am in a group, I am against a wall, sitting in a chair, or my back up to a table. I always try to give a front view. I have two older sisters who are 5'7" and weigh over 300 pounds. I am 4'11" and weigh 105 pounds. In my family, the fact that I was short and thin caused more jealousy and problems than my having scoliosis.

I was in and out of the hospital for two years. I had my spinal fusion at a medical center quite a distance from my home. Both my parents worked and were unable to visit me often. The hospital became my home and I learned to love it there. While in the hospital I wore a body cast that extended from the top of my head down to my toes. After surgery, I had to be flat on my back for 12 months. The cast was changed periodically and I gradually moved to an upright position in a wheel chair. When the cast was removed permanently, I had to learn to walk again with crutches. Following that, I wore a back brace until I was about 15 years old.

In high school I was a majorette and my uniform never quite fit me right. I was embarrassed to wear it. The belt never hung right. There are a lot of things I can do but won't because I can't find the right clothes to wear. I'll never overcome having scoliosis because I don't think other people accept it. It just drives me crazy when people stare. My mother was always saying to me, 'Sharon, everyone has something wrong, but it is not always visible.' In fact, I remember when I started dating and going to dances or parties and I would be so self-conscious. When it came time to dance, I'd get tense because that meant my partner would have to put his hand on my body. As a result, I became an expert at *fast* dancing. It was something I could do alone—without anyone touching me.

I met my husband, David, when I was 16. I didn't tell him about scoliosis at first. When we started getting serious I knew I would have to tell him, but my family beat me to it. I think they thought they would scare him away. But, David never mentioned anything to me. Months later when he gave me his fraternity pin, I brought up the subject. When I started to tell him, he said, 'Stop, I already know.' I've had this feeling for many years, that if the situation were reversed and it was he who had scoliosis, I don't think I would feel the same way toward him as he feels toward me. I don't know if I would marry a man with the same condition that I have.

I don't like myself. I feel that the personality I developed—being outgoing, happy-go-lucky and bubbly, is a cover-up to make it easier for others to accept me for what I am. If I were mousy and quiet with scoliosis, where would it get me? I never forget for a minute that I have scoliosis. How do I stand a chance when my mother has saved all the bills from my surgery and still keeps my brace down in her basement. She still refers to me as 'Poor Sharon, how I pity you.' She'll never say, 'Look at what you've accomplished, or how far you've come.'

Scoliosis is like a burden that once shared becomes lighter. Talking to others helps relieve some of the anxiety. I think about surgery, that it could reduce my curve from 92 degrees to about 60 degrees. I was told that with surgery I could be 2″ taller with a 30 per cent improvement in the curvature. Just think, I could buy a new wardrobe and maybe even like my body again. I am finally happy with what I am doing. Besides having four children to keep me hopping, I jog, bowl once a week, play racquet ball two times a week, and work part-time as a teacher's aide. Perhaps when my family is a bit more self-sufficient, I'll consider a second surgery. Right now, I'm just taking one day at a time."

BRENDA

Born: 1949

"I remember my mom and sister trying to wash my hair with my body cast on and me flat on my back. I couldn't sit up, so I would have to be laid across the width of the bed with my head hanging over buckets of water. Everyone was wet when we were finished."

Brenda was born in 1949. She is married and has one daughter. Her scoliosis was detected when she came down with the flu. Her mother took her to see a doctor at which time he diagnosed scoliosis and put her through a year of exercise. About a year later, at the age of 12 he said surgery was indicated because the curve was progressing rapidly. Brenda was also on the swim team at school and became very self-conscious because one hip was much higher than the other.

"I really feel fortunate about the outcome of my surgery. The people close to me, my mom, dad, sister and two brothers, deserve all the credit for my positive feelings. I was bedridden for six months following my fusion. I was totally dependent on my family. My parents put me in our sun room on the main floor of the house so I would feel part of the family. I had an in-service teacher come to my house during that six-month period so I wouldn't fall behind in my school work. My mother would always fix beautiful and colorful trays of food. There was always something to keep my morale up.

I remember my mom and sister trying to wash my hair. I couldn't sit up, so I would have to be laid across the width of the bed with my head hanging over buckets of water which were used to wash my hair. Most of the time, everyone was wet when we finished. I also remember my older brother helping me stand upright after the six-month period of bed rest ended.

I had no idea that scoliosis was genetic. Of course, I don't think knowing that would have changed my mind from having a child of my own. I delivered my daughter, now seven, by natural childbirth because I didn't want anyone near my back with a shot.

I am proud to talk about having scoliosis. My memories and experiences have made me stronger both mentally and physically. Hopefully, my daughter will not develop scoliosis. But, if she does, I'll be there for her as my family and friends were for me."

DORENE

Born: 1952

"I was approximately 5'10" tall when I was braced at 14 years of age. Given the combination of towering over 90% of my classmates plus wearing a brace, made for a large difference in my social life."

Doreen was born in 1952. She is married and has one child. Her scoliosis was discovered at the age of nine and was followed for three years by an orthopedic surgeon. At the age of 12, Doreen's mother expressed concern to the doctor that her daughter's condition seemed to be worsening. Doreen remarked that he looked at the X-ray, patted her on the shoulder and patted her mother's hand saying, "She's got a pretty face, get her a good tailor, and she'll be fine."

"That shattering advice flabbergasted my mother and we started to make rounds of local doctors for other advice. End of tale? Wrong! We saw seven orthopods all of whom indicated that surgery wasn't necessary. This was in 1966.

My emotional life changed very little at the age of 10 or 11 because I didn't realize it was a *problem*. After I was braced, however, things changed. I knew I was crooked, but because my major curve was low on my spine, my appearance was OK! We finally ended up with a doctor in another state for bracing treatment. However, by age 14 most of my growth had been completed and I eventually went to another major center for surgery. Bracing affected me negatively and some of that negative image remains today. Putting a very noticeable metal appliance on a teenager, during the important adolescent formative years, has to have some long-lasting effects.

Today, I am 5'10" in height. I was just about this height when I was braced at 14. Given the combination of towering over 90% of my classmates *plus* wearing the brace, made for a large difference in my social life.

I am by profession a social worker, but presently I am unemployed staying at home to care for my daughter. I exercise twice a week for about three hours, sew, knit, walk, read, paint and houseclean. All my limitations are self-imposed. I won't, for example, horseback ride or ice skate for fear of falling and hurting my back."

ELAINE

Born: 1950

"The hardest thing is knowing what your limitations are and whether you should push ahead, or rest."

Elaine was born in 1950, had a spinal fusion at the age of 13, which required her to miss a year from school and to be bedridden for 10 months. Her mother, sisters, and grandparents also have scoliosis. These experiences she feels, contributed to her being a loner. Elaine is married and has no children.

"When I was a teenager, I felt that everyone saw my raised hip. Since my surgery, I don't think about it any more. I still have a sensitive feeling in my upper and lower back around the surgical scar area. Often this becomes more pronounced around my period or with weather changes. Off and on, I have stiffness in my hips. This I find is somewhat relieved with aspirin.

I am a librarian. I do a lot of walking and climbing stairs. I find myself limited to quiet activities such as reading, sewing, needlepoint, cooking, refinishing furniture, swimming and certain specific muscle strengthening exercises. Limitations have been placed on me with regard to "impact sports" such as tennis and running.

The hardest thing is knowing what your limitations are and whether you should push ahead, or rest. I find that the discomfort I am having is nagging rather than incapacitating. I manage to override the discomfort."

SYLVIA

Born: 1931

*"Scoliosis has definitely had an affect on my life.
I feel that it makes me try harder."*

Sylvia was born in 1931. She is married with two grown children. Her father had rheumatoid arthritis and a fused spine. One of her cousins was diagnosed as having arthritis with scoliosis. The women in her family were all very round shouldered. Sylvia also remembers a cousin that wore a brace for a couple of years but never required surgery.

"I was discharged from the care of my orthopedic surgeon when I was engaged to be married at age 18. Everything was fine for another 10–12 years. At age 30, I started having back problems. Most of the pain was in my neck more than anywhere else. I usually have to lie down with support for my neck. While working and keeping busy, I'm OK. It is when I am sitting and relaxing that additional support is needed. I went for neurological tests that showed I have a degenerative disc problem. I also have extreme pain in my lower back. My problems seem to be a little scoliosis and a little arthritis.

My experience with scoliosis and a spinal fusion at the age of 11 was a fairly positive one. As a result it has left me with a great deal of compassion and understanding for people with physical problems. During my 4–6 week hospital stay as a child, I was bedridden. Following the hospital I went to a convalescent home with children who had all kinds of conditions. All were bedridden. I couldn't really feel sorry for myself because everyone there had either the same problem or one that was worse. I had to go back to the hospital for a second step of the surgery. When I finally came home after a total of nine months, I was wearing a brace day and night for 6–8 months longer.

I don't think scoliosis should make anyone an invalid in any way. It doesn't mean that you can do things better than anyone else, but there certainly isn't any reason why a person with scoliosis shouldn't feel that they are every bit as good as anyone else! Scoliosis has definitely had an affect on my life. I feel that it makes me try harder."

MARION

Born: 1944

"Probably the most important factor in adjustment, productivity and happiness in life is not a disability itself, but rather the attitudes and expectations of close family and friends."

Marion was born in 1944 with congenital scoliosis. She is widowed and the mother of two children.

"I was born with scoliosis. It was very severe and my mother was advised to put me in an institution. There wasn't anything that could be done, she was told, and I wasn't expected to live very long. The statement was made at the time, that I would never sit, walk or raise my head off the pillow." Because I was born with scoliosis, there was never any separation. I can't say that at age twelve I developed scoliosis, because it didn't happen that way.

I had my first spinal surgery at the age of six at a hospital where I had to stay for 13 months. I went in during the first grade and came out when I was in the second grade. When my mother came to pick me up, I looked like something out of the African pictures. I look real skeletal in pictures that were taken of me then because my weight had dropped quite low. Here I was, a kid my mother hadn't seen in 13 months.

My mother, at that time, had no support. We left the hospital, suitcase in hand to ride by bus, subways, and taxis to get back to my home state. When I was 11 years old, my mother remarried. Her new husband, who eventually adopted me, came into this marriage with two children from his first marriage. My mother also had a child from this marriage. So, I went from just my mother and me to a new father and 3 brothers and sisters.

I learned a lot of skills in the hospital like shutting off my feelings. I had to be very strong, because that was what I thought was expected of me. While in the hospital I had a lot of different treatments: a cellulose jacket and casts with turnbuckles and traction. I guess what I resent most about my memories of the hospital stay was I never was allowed to get my own sense of privacy. I have always been exposed to other people asking me to take off my clothes. I have never been allowed to have my body all to myself.

I got married at the age of 18. Due to my mixed up childhood, I really had no good role model to follow how a marriage should be and how people got along, solved their problems, and planned for the future. I didn't really have a good relationship with my husband, but we cared for each other. He filed for divorce eventually due to all of our problems.

When I was young, I was told I couldn't have children. That is all one has to say to me—that I can't do something and then I will go about doing it. I had problems delivering my children. There just wasn't enough room. I was 4½ feet tall and weighed 80 pounds. My son weighed 7 pounds, 13 ounces. There just wasn't room for both of us. My parenting skills were horrible. I won't know for a while how my kids turned out. Right now my daughter is boy crazy, which I believe is normal. My son is extremely attractive. Fortunately, I have real good-looking kids. They do not have scoliosis.

I am extremely uncomfortable in social situations and try to avoid them. I am a very good worker and a very poor socializer. It took me a long time to find out what I like to do. Currently, I am getting a master's degree in counseling. This activity is serving as both educational and recreational. For the first time, last year, I got a handicapped parking sticker for my car to park closer to my classes at the university. I am not uncomfortable with that, but it was something I really had to do. I am finding it increasingly difficult to carry the vacuum cleaner up the stairs of our town house. My kids just have to help me more. When the weather gets cold, I have trouble breathing. I haven't cut out anything I am presently doing, I just keep doing more. I also complain more.

Probably the most important factor in adjustment, productivity, and happiness in life is not a disability itself, but rather the attitudes and expectations of close family and friends. My recommendations for anyone with scoliosis is to *choose* their family of origin carefully—which of course, cannot be done! But, I believe that this factor is as important, if not more so, than scoliosis itself."

CHAPTER **4**

Learning to Live With It . . . Or Is There Life After Scoliosis?

To have or not to have surgery is a tough decision to make whether one is an adult, or the parent of a child. It takes a long mental process which includes getting through feelings of despair and anger, "why me" attitudes, information sorting, anxiety, until finally an awareness or acceptance is reached. The doctor and patient must build a bond of trust working together to reach a suitable course of treatment that is based on the premise of improving the quality of life.

The way we perceive ourselves is difficult to change. But, has scoliosis had an effect on what direction our lives take—one's choice of careers, lifestyle or even the choice of a mate? The following are twelve personal interviews with men and women choosing to have surgery as adults: Liz, Jessica, Jane, Louise, Leslie, Bob, Pamela, Patricia, Jerry, Melissa, Margaret-Ann, Kim.

LIZ

Born: 1947

"Before deciding to have surgery, I lost 40 percent of my breathing capacity and I was losing height. I wanted to stop the progression, prevent further pain, and avoid the side effects such as respiratory problems."

Liz was born in 1947. She is married and the mother of two children.

"My mother noticed one day that my back was abnormal when we were in the department store trying on bras. We immediately went home to call the doctor who then referred us to an orthopedic surgeon. The doctor prescribed a brace which I wore through high school. I dated very little in high school. My mother thought that as a result of my wearing a brace that I became cold, unfeeling and didn't like to be touched. She told me this later on. She also felt people viewed me as a cripple. My feeling is, if that's the way people are, then it's their loss. Granted, I don't have a sparkling personality—but, if you get all involved with boys in high school, you'll never make it through school and college.

Before I decided to have surgery as an adult, I had lost 40 percent of my breathing capacity. My projected height (determined by the arm spread) was 5'6". I was 5'3" before surgery and now measure 5'5". I had decided to have surgery to stop the progression, prevent further pain, and stop further side effects such as respiratory problems. My curve was 75 degrees.

I was a real pain in the hospital. One night I rolled over and thought I heard the rods snap. I got hysterical. The doctor on staff ordered X-rays. Fortunately nothing was wrong.

When my husband first saw me in the hospital after surgery, he was scared of me. I tried to pull him in bed with me, but he just wouldn't. He was afraid he would hurt me. Actually, I was feeling pretty good and pretty anxious to become active again after a two-week bed rest. After the body cast was put on, my husband discovered sex was terrific. He found he could put his whole body weight on me and I wouldn't mind.

Before I went into the hospital, I had cut my hair and had it permed so that it wouldn't be a problem. After a week and a half the nurses decided to have it washed. They tried propping me up on the bed and putting garbage bags on the floor to catch the water. The Sunday before I was to get my body cast on, I wanted my hair washed again. By now they had their technique down to a science. When I was taken down to the operating room for the cast, I was nice and clean. Now, imagine getting a cast put on that goes up over your shoulders and around your body with all this wet plaster, you can guess the outcome. I came back to my room looking like I had a helmet on. The first thing the nurse said was, 'You are going to get your hair washed.'

When the cast was cut down, I went back to work as a substitute teacher. The doctor told me I had no limitations. Now, looking back, my advice to an adult or child with scoliosis is to get it checked. Talk to people who are dealing with it. People who find out for the first time that they have scoliosis tend to get bent out of shape. Find out for yourself . . . there is life after scoliosis."

JESSICA

Born: 1957

"I lived on the Army base with my husband while recovering from my spinal fusion. Developing a positive attitude about myself was absolutely necessary especially when the guys look at every female who walks by."

Jessica was born in 1957. Her scoliosis was discovered by accident in 1974 when she was taken to the doctor for an X-ray due to pneumonia.

"I always felt something was wrong with my back because my pediatrician always traced my spine with his fingers during school check-ups. When I was eleven or twelve years old and taking Hunter Safety Class, the instructor constantly straightened my head while I was shooting in the prone position. Bracing was not recommended for me because judging from my bone age, I was too old for it to do any good. Surgery was not even suggested as a possibility.

The decision to have surgery was made after I was married. My mom really helped me through it. She came and stayed with me when I came home from the hospital. I really needed the help and support. I was teaching, taking care of my mother-in-law, and dealing with my own surgery. I feel that I have gone through more at my age than most people go through in a lifetime. As a result, I have developed greater patience and understanding to help others through their medical problems. I feel that this surgery helped me gain insight that I did not have before. It also taught me that when you are going against nature you lose something of yourself. I want to help someone else gain back their control and dignity.

Pain was the reason that I decided to have the surgery. I couldn't garden and do the things that I normally loved to do. My husband, Bill, had to do much of my work for me. While recuperating from the surgery, I had made up my mind to be in the best possible shape that I could. I felt very cramped in the body cast—like I couldn't breathe. I wanted my muscles to be in good shape when the cast came off, so I joined a health spa, played racquet ball, and kept myself in good condition. I lived on the Army base with my husband while recovering from my spinal fusion. Developing a positive attitude about myself was absolutely necessary especially when the guys on the base would look at every female that walked by.

The cast itself, was my biggest problem. I didn't like the way other people looked at me. Sometimes I felt like I *was* handicapped. My husband was really great to me. My family, on the other hand, was somewhat over-protective. I knew I couldn't let my dad see me until everything about me was up to his standards. When he finally glanced at my back after the cast was off and saw the scar, he remarked, 'It's not that bad.'

I guess, through my growing up years, I felt a little jealousy toward my younger sister. She was born with half of a cleft palate and a bit of a hare lip. She needed a lot of work done to her mouth and received a lot of attention when we were young and growing up in the same house. She needed it done, I didn't begrudge her, but here I am with scoliosis and in the need of surgery. I guess that I wished someone had paid attention to my back.

When I had my second cast made, I had my breasts enclosed. The first cast made my breasts droopy and hang so low and limp that I looked like a native from another society. I also developed a herniated disc while in my first cast. It was so disappointing to me. I had to have complete bed rest. For some reason I was very relaxed about sex while in the body cast. I just felt psychologically better and safer—isn't that strange? When I came home from the hospital, I was afraid that our first attempt at lovemaking in the bodycast would make me laugh and I would start hurting. But, it was great!

Now that I am all done with the casts, I want to look great! I want people to look at me and say—'Boy, is she sharp!' I want to look my best all of the time. I don't think I felt that way before.

I don't think I'm unique or unusual. But, I do believe it's very important to maintain and indeed perpetuate a positive outlook on life. I've never been one to put limits on my abilities, so when my scoliosis became constantly painful, I was really upset. When I learned that a spinal fusion would help, I jumped at the chance. I don't want to *ever* be limited by my physical condition."

JANE

Born: 1951

"I am one of those kids who was detected early, released at 18 and told my back would never get worse."

Jane was born in 1951. Her scoliosis was detected in the 7th grade and treated by observation and periodic X-rays. A brace was discussed by the doctor treating Jane, but she decided against using it. Her scoliosis was not very noticeable at this time.

"I am one of those kids who was detected early in the schools, who was released at age 18 and told my back would never get worse. At the age of 27 I had surgery.

During my recovery period from my fusion, I spent three months in bed in a nursing home because I didn't want to move back home for the care that was needed. I had to push myself to make all the necessary arrangements, because it was my choice to do this alone. I do feel satisfied with my decision to have the surgery as an adult, choosing my doctor and the course of treatment suited for my needs.

I have been an artist all my life. I was on disability and received benefits during my eight month recovery period from my fusion. I find that I do have limitations especially with my friends. I tire long before they do and usually get very irritable.

My sister also had a spinal fusion, but as a child. I always had difficulty dealing with the attention she received. I did finally see a counselor for about six months regarding this issue.

My leisure time activities, after I get home from work and in between studying and working on my graduate studies which lasts until 11:30 P.M., consist of swimming during the summer approximately 1 hour a day for 5 days a week."

LOUISE

Born: 1935

"In paraphrasing the words of an old song that sort of winds up my feelings about scoliosis, I'd say, "You've got to accentuate the positive, eliminate the negative, and don't mess with what's in between."

Louise was born in 1935. She is divorced and the mother of one son. Her scoliosis was detected at the age of eleven by her mother who had noticed one shoulder blade protruding and one shoulder higher than the other.

"At the same time that my mother noticed something wrong, I was also experiencing back pain. We went to the family physician for an opinion. It was there that my condition was diagnosed as scoliosis. I heard the doctor tell my mother that I should go to a hospital that was located quite a distance from my home. I knew I'd be away from my family and panic set in.

I finally did go to a hospital at the age of 12 and was suspended by my chin and wrapped in a complete body cast from the top of my head to my knees. A bar was placed between my knees to facilitate moving me as a patient. It was also used to prevent the cast from splitting in two. After the cast dried, wedges were cut on both sides and turnbuckles (a screw device used to add more pressure) was inserted. The doctor would come in every two days, turn the turnbuckle screws to tighten it a bit more. The purpose was to obtain maximum correction prior to surgery. If this was possible, and the correction could be stabilized for a month, then I would have a spinal fusion. In my particular case, the correction was not enough to warrant surgery. I was written off, released and sent home.

The years to follow, 13 on up, were hard on my emotions and shattered self-image. I became very shy, secluded and withdrawn. Clothes never fit right and though my dear mom tried to have them made by a seamstress, she always wanted to pad my shoulders to make them even. The hemlines, too, were always put up crooked to make them appear even. At that time, I felt like an ugly stuffed old clown that was on display for everyone to see. Remarks from peers naturally came, including being called the *Hunchback of Notre Dame*. That would hurt any youngster being called names, but it especially hurts when you know you can't do anything about it.

Things changed for me at about age 18. My sister came to me with an article that was taken from a magazine. The article explained a new technique for scoliosis which consisted of the insertion of a metal rod along the spinal column and attached to the top and bottom vertebra. Adjustments were made to get as much correction as possible. When correction was obtained, the rod was tightened and left to remain there to support the spine and prevent it from getting worse. No bone graft was used for a spinal fusion. Through correspondence I made arrangements to see the doctor. He checked me over and said because of my bone age, the results would not be as great as they would have been had I come sooner. But, he did see some play in the bone and curve and said he'd be willing to give it a try. I agreed to have the surgery in 1954.

The surgery involved going through my chest cage, moving my heart and cutting out five ribs. After surgery, I learned to walk all over again. I was in bed for a month. The young doctor that assisted my doctor in surgery encouraged me to take the first few steps. What a glorious day! I stood so straight and tall. Even though I wasn't completely straight, I felt like a princess.

Since that surgery, I spent the next 25 years feeling that I had done the best thing ever for myself. Over the years, however, the degree of my curvature has increased, the rod has become loose, and further rotation set in.

I was married for 23 years and just recently divorced my husband. When my husband and I were dating, he was the one who wanted to marry. I didn't want to get married because I felt I didn't want to give this burden to anyone. I just kept refusing. He just kept asking. Eventually, I agreed to marry him. We had many good years together. I did have an uneventful pregnancy and now have a 15-year-old son. I've done everything anyone else could do, even as far as shoveling snow, driving, working in various office situations and doing my own housework."

With the absence of scoliosis, Louise felt she would have gone on to greater heights, motivating herself to go to college, or to attain a higher job position. "I feel that I was held back especially in the job market due to my scoliosis. I've had a lot of problems obtaining work since my divorce and worsening condition. Recently, I went to the Vocational Rehabilitation Service for an evaluation. I had X-rays, blood tests, the works. Their doctors turned me down as "unemployable" because of scoliosis. On an X-ray the loosened rod can be seen. They think it is something that could cause a big medical problem for a potential employer.

Clothing is so important to a person with scoliosis. My advice is to find clothes that fit properly and don't worry about size. If your clothes are put together and coordinated so that you look and feel comfortable, that's all that matters. Furthermore, you are the only one who knows. To paraphrase the words of an old song, I feel it sort of winds up my feelings about scoliosis: *You have to accentuate the positive, eliminate the negative, and don't mess with what's in between."*

LESLIE

Born: 1951

"I really don't expect any change from my forthcoming surgery except maybe I'll be a more pleasant person. I won't be so nervous about whether I'll be paralyzed or die. Little things like that!"

Leslie was born in 1951. Her scoliosis was diagnosed at the age of 13 and didn't really cause much of a problem until around age 28. Leslie is single.

'Did you ever notice how people with scoliosis always take a lot upon themselves? Maybe that is why our backs are weak—we are work horses!' When my scoliosis was discovered at age 13, I didn't even know what the word meant.

In 1980, after 13 years of not giving any thought to my back, I am told by an orthopedic surgeon that my back is curved enough to require surgery. I started to seek medical attention after catching a glimpse of a public service announcement about scoliosis on television. This was either an act of *God* or a twist of fate because I rarely watch TV. The announcement told of the dangers of scoliosis and listed Scoliosis Centers for further information.

My mom and dad were divorced when I was five years old. My mom raised me and my sister alone. Now my mom has a little business that she has owned for about nine years. I did graduate from college as an elementary school teacher. But, teaching was definitely not for me. I now work in the store with my mother. Occasionally, my little niece stays with us. I tell her a story about the large picture of an old woman carrying a heavy bucket of water in one hand. She bends to one side because it is such a heavy burden. I tell her that I am the reincarnation of that woman in the picture and that explains the reason my back is crooked today due to the continued carrying of so many buckets of water to my cottage.

When I went to the doctor to see my X-rays, I couldn't believe they were mine. The only way I was certain they were, was because I forgot to take off my necklace and I could see it in the X-ray.

I really don't expect any change from this surgery except maybe I'll be a more pleasant person. I won't be so nervous about whether I'll be paralyzed or die. Little things like that! I have been feeling very anxious and tense due to my forthcoming surgery. I do not talk much about these fears and future problems because I'm afraid it will turn people off.

Actually, I think I am fairly straight now. I am not humped over. Occasionally, someone will ask me if I have a stiff neck, but they never comment about my back. My hair is very long and does cover most of my back, so no one can really tell.

Perhaps after surgery I will have an award-winning story about my experience with scoliosis. The plot will go something like this: a handsome doctor meets patient to set her straight. They get married and live happily ever after. The story will be called, *Love in a Body Cast* or *Romantic Encounters of the Plaster Kind*. (laughter)

BOB

Born: 1952

"I am always testing for limitations. But, I found out one by one, that I could still do the things I wanted to do like basketball, racquetball, and water skiing. I went winter camping in Northern Canada six months after I was out of my cast."

Bob was born in 1952. He had a spinal fusion at the age of 27. His scoliosis was detected at the age of 18. Bob is one of five children. He feels that his surgery and that of his brother helped to bring the family closer together.

"Both my older brother, Al, and myself had spinal fusions. He had his surgery at the age of 39, and I had mine at 27. My brother just wants to forget about the whole thing, while I really don't mind talking about it. I feel now, that the short period I was laid up was just temporary, and now things are back to normal. I kind of view this like a broken arm or something temporary like that.

Before I had surgery, people would notice my scoliosis and as a result I would try to stand up straight. When I see pictures of myself, I'll notice how stiff I am sitting, or how awkward I look at doing certain things. Generally, most people do not realize the fact that I have scoliosis.

Having scoliosis surgery has made me try to test my limitations. I realized that I would have to live with certain things, so I set out to prove to myself that I could do anything I wanted. One by one, as I tested myself with what I liked to do like basketball, racquetball, water skiing, I found out there was no problem. I went winter camping in Northern Canada six months after I was out of my cast. I was still waiting for that limitation. One winter I went cross country camping in the snow in the back woods of Canada wearing snow shoes and carrying a 70 pound toboggan while walking for miles. It went down to 20 below zero. I wouldn't recommend it for everyone, but for me, it proved that my back did not present a problem through this whole thing. My fear of limitation proved to be an imaginary one. Also, my job as a photographer is a physically demanding one—setting up scaffolding, taking it down, carrying the cases up and down and sometimes fighting severe winds in the process.

I knew I had scoliosis when I was 18 years old. I wore a Milwaukee Brace for a short while. I found that at that time I really avoided talking about it and even ignored that there was a problem. I always thought of scoliosis as the other guy's problem. When I had my curve checked again, it was determined that it was 65 degrees and I needed surgery. I was scared, but I knew I had to make a decision. I began to research scoliosis, reading medical books, talking to doctors, and anyone else I could find. I decided to have the surgery out-of-state at the major scoliosis center where my brother had his spinal fusion.

I was in the hospital for 10 days. I planned to drive back home in a rented car. But, my mom and dad decided it wasn't a good idea so they came with their car and we drove back together. That was really nice. However, my surgery threw everything off in my life. I planned to return to California, where I was living, two weeks after surgery, thinking I could take care of myself. I ended up staying with my parents for two years. In between, I went back to California to move everything back here. Now I have a job nearby that I really enjoy.

Surgery makes one vulnerable. All of a sudden the tables are turned and here, we, who were the once healthy individuals, are in need of help. Being vulnerable, being limited in what one can do, and being discriminated against are all the things that a handicapped person has to go through on a day-to-day basis. Fortunately, it is only temporary and we quickly get back to where we were before.

I would consider any of the emotional problems as important as any of the physical. Personally, what I tried to do was disprove a lot of fears by going out and actually doing what I feared most. I tried to keep a sense of humor throughout the whole experience and not get too serious about it all. When one takes things too seriously one tends to get depressed and not think clearly about the whole situation. There is not too much I feel we can do for the physical end of the surgery for scoliosis. But I feel we can always lend some emotional support by listening to what these people have to say and letting them talk about what is really bothering them. So many times we are really only half listening or trying to get our equal time back in. From my experience, I feel one of the best things we could give to a person with scoliosis is not something we could run and buy in the stores, but something we all have to give. That something is support and attention."

PAMELA

Born: 1953

"Not anyone or anything could have changed my mind or outlook about what needed to be done. I feel that having surgery was the best thing I could have done for myself."

Pamela was born in 1953. She had her scoliosis checked by a doctor when she was 13 years old. He took X-rays and told her to return in a year. When she returned after the year, he checked her and told her to come back in two years. At this time she was 16 years old. No bracing was recommended. Pamela was under the impression that once one stops growing, it wouldn't get worse.

"I could tell something was wrong because my pants always needed one leg shortened more than the other. However, I felt that the curvature was something I could live with. But, realizing it was getting worse encouraged me to take action and learn more about the condition.

My mother has scoliosis and hers has progressed noticeably over the years. She is now 57 years old and probably started out with a curve similar to mine. No treatment was recommended for her curvature. She stands up straight, but she is very short waisted and her rib hump is noticeable and prominent.

I decided to have surgery in 1979 at the age of 26. I knew that I was making the right decision. I just had to look at my mother. My two sisters also have mild degrees of curvature. Of my mother's six children, I have it the worst. Both my parents were with me on the day of my surgery. They were very supportive. I stayed in the hospital for two weeks and went back to my parent's house and rested for four weeks. After six weeks, I went back to work at the hospital where I analyze blood for the blood bank. There was a stipulation that I couldn't lift anything more than 10 pounds. I did have to go to health services where I obtained a letter from my supervisor stating my job didn't require me to do lifting.

While in the hospital, my present boyfriend came to see me every day. I had just met him a week prior to my going into the hospital. Now, here I am going in for surgery, planning on wearing a body cast for the next eight to nine months and thinking, 'That's the last he's going to want of me.' But, I was surprised at his response. He told me that he wanted to continue to see me and he was thinking that I wouldn't want to see him. He remarked, 'I liked you before because you were an interesting person, and now I still want to see you.' That worked out really well. We spent a lot of time together just getting to know one another.

Not anyone or anything could have changed my mind or outlook about what needed to be done. I researched the subject at the university medical library. I looked up a book on possible complications and how the surgical procedure was done. I wanted to know everything. I feel very positive and better about myself now. I feel I am a more open person.

One week after my cast change, I went downhill skiing up north with my boyfriend. We skied for two solid days. He was having trouble keeping up with me. I thought I wouldn't be able to ski very well afterwards, but it didn't cause any problems. Prior to my surgery I skied a great deal in Colorado. It's all in the knees anyway. I also went cross-country skiing and rollerskating in my body cast. *I, of course, wouldn't recommend taking up the sport following surgery, if one has never practiced this before!* I did fall once or twice, but not hard. I am a daring person, anyway. I like to test my limitations.

After my cast came off, I felt a little stiff. I didn't feel great right away. But, after about a week, I went to a health spa and exercised gently, avoiding any bending or twisting. I swam, doing just the breast and back stroke. I really felt quite physically fit. I feel that having surgery was the best thing I could have done for myself. My back looks very straight now, and I don't have to worry about my curve getting worse."

PATRICIA

Born: 1953

"I was married about two years when I decided to make an appointment with the orthopedic surgeon. I thought it would be a good idea to know about problems or precautions before getting pregnant."

Patricia was born in 1953. She was 14 years old when she wore a Milwaukee Brace. The brace was worn 23 hours a day to start. Then, the last year of her treatment she wore it just to bed. Supposedly, bracing stabilized the curve. So, all the years from graduation from high school, until the time Patricia got married, she thought everything was OK!

"Jim and I were married about two years, when I decided to make an appointment with the orthopedic surgeon. I thought it would be a good idea to know about any problems or precautions I should take before getting pregnant. I brought previous X-rays with me and they were compared with present ones. The doctor felt that I should have surgery before I even decide to *get* pregnant. My degree of curvature increased to 82 degrees by the time I was scheduled for surgery. I also knew I had lost height because when I was measured before surgery I was 5'7½" and my driver's license read, 5'8½". When I found out that I had to wear a back brace as a child I was *crushed*. When I found out that I had to have surgery, I was a *mess!*

A week after my appointment with the doctor, Jim and I made another appointment for a consultation together. The doctor explained the surgical procedure he would use, the risks involved, and the prognosis. He left it up to us to decide. Neither of us thought there was any decision to make. If it needs to be done, then do it! We told my family that evening. My mother cried! A mother just hates to see her own kids go through this, especially when she thought it was taken care of the first time.

I had my surgery in March, 1979, and wore a body cast until December. I was in the hospital for two weeks and home for two months before going back to work. Personally, I feel my husband had the rough end. I kept putting responsibility on him. After two months, when I returned to work as a secretary, I brought a pillow to prop up in my chair. I managed quite well.

I am very critical of my appearance. I am extra careful always checking my back view in the mirror. When I was younger, I always wore my hair real long thinking it would help camouflage my back. But, one can't be 40, 50 or 60 years old and still expect to have hair flowing down one's back. My school clothes were always slanted because my hips were out of line. I remember wearing flowered skirts as a kid with belts. I think there is a social stigma about perfection. In public places you don't want to feel different and you certainly don't want people staring at you.

Scoliosis has not really changed my life at all. I don't have high aspirations and I'm not goal oriented. It doesn't take much to make me happy. My husband makes me very happy and I think that is very important. I am not obsessed with materialism. I think that it is important to feel secure in one's personal relationships and constantly build upon them. With my upbringing and support and closeness of my family, I don't think I would feel any different with the absence of scoliosis. Families play an important role in influencing the outcomes of our lives.

Jim and I discussed my having scoliosis when we were dating. I wouldn't have been able to get married if something that major wasn't discussed first. However, timing is important when one is really attracted to someone. One doesn't want to scare off a good prospect too early in the game. When one gets to the point of becoming more serious, then that person has the right to know and vice versa. After all, that other person may have things he may wish not to talk about either!"

Postscript: Patricia delivered a 10 pound 12 ounce, 23 inch long baby girl by C-section. Mother, daughter, and father are all doing fine!

JERRY

Born: 1944

"I love acting on the stage. I feel that with the absence of scoliosis there would be some different parts I would try. My friends will occasionally joke about my scoliosis and tell me I'd make a good Quasimodo."

Jerry was born in 1944 and was 16 years old when his parents decided to take him to the doctor to have his curvature checked. "It was an emotional experience for me, probably one of the most difficult experiences in my youth. The doctor told me that to correct this curvature I would have to have surgery and be in a body cast for my senior year in high school. Certainly, I didn't want to be in a cast and miss any part of my senior year. It is very easy to look back now, from an older point of view and say that 16 to 17 or 12 to 13 is not so significant a span of years when you think of the rest of your life. Now, looking back, my curvature has increased about one degree per year since I was 16. Today, I have a lot more concerns than just that of missing my senior year.

Scoliosis was discovered when I was playing baseball. One of my friends said to me, 'How come one side of your back is bigger than the other?' That was all I needed to hear. I pointed this out to my parents. At some point we discussed it and I was taken to a doctor. My father had muscular dystrophy. The symptoms got worse in his mid 20's. Things were very rough for my mother who eventually had to take care of my father until his death. I didn't grow up in a warm, loving family relationship, especially where my father was concerned. My father was an engineer and an efficiency expert. I enjoyed getting away from home because there was too much of a burden there. I had to do things for him. For example, not only did I have to cut the grass which was a normal request for a kid, but he checked on how fast I could do it. He believed in saving time, eliminating waste, being fast and measuring how good.

At 18 years old I was called into the draft. I remember going back to the doctor that examined me at age 16 to get a letter saying that I had scoliosis. He also wrote that my father had muscular dystrophy and it may be related. I also had poor vision and wore contact lenses. Finally, added to that, he put that I had flat feet. I thought that bad eyes and flat feet would have been enough to keep me out of the service, but to that I added scoliosis.

I was married in 1967. I remember talking to my wife before, telling her that I had scoliosis. All the while I was thinking, 'Well, Jerry, that's going to be the end of the relationship.' Surprisingly enough, it didn't phase her at all. She has been the best thing that has happened to me!

Scoliosis may have had some effect on me as far as being more family oriented. My two boys are getting older and I want to do things with them, have a pleasant family life, have grandchildren and all that good kind of stuff. My family life is a lot more important to me now than when we first got married when my mind was on just teaching and maybe someday becoming a principal. Somehow that doesn't seem all that important now.

I think that I have a reasonably positive self-image. Other than the appearance of my back, I think I look OK! It bothers me to have that defect and I wish I didn't have it, but it doesn't stop me from all that I like to do. I love acting on the stage. I mean, talk about having people look at you—stage acting is pretty straight forward looking! I feel that with the absence of scoliosis, there would be some different parts I would want to try. My friends will sometimes joke about my having scoliosis and tell me that I'd make a good Quasimodo. I would like to play King Richard III. I sure would look at him with a different perspective today than I would have several years ago.

I am really uncomfortable wearing a tight shirt that shows the lines of my back. If it doesn't fit well after it has been washed, I won't wear it anymore. I realize that I can't hide scoliosis, but I do try to minimize the appearance of my back by wearing loose fitting clothes, jackets and sweaters. I do not look at this forthcoming surgery as being the end all to my troubles. I do know that without having it done, it would begin to involve internal organs, be harder to correct, involve more pain and backaches and perhaps shorten my life expectancy. I think that having scoliosis gives one a great deal of insight into understanding oneself. In the long run, who knows, I may have been better off waiting for this surgery as an adult."

MELISSA

Born: 1943

"Scoliosis has never stopped me from doing anything that I've ever wanted to do. My biggest hope with surgery is that it will stop the progression and any further problems."

Melissa was born in 1943. Her mother has scoliosis and encouraged her to consider surgery as an adult. Her mother always thought that Melissa's scoliosis was caused by a fall she had when she was 12 years old.

"I have never considered scoliosis a handicap. I think that anyone who does is misleading themselves. My curve is now 96 degrees, so it isn't a slight curvature by any means. However, it has never stopped me from doing anything that I've ever wanted to do. I bowl, snowmobile, square dance, golf, do yard work and hang wallpaper.

My mother is the one who led me to have this surgery. We came to the Scoliosis Clinic to have our backs checked together. All along, we have thought that my back was the worst. But, now when I look at my mother's, I see hers is the worst. She now feels that at the age of 63 nothing more can be done for her.

The day I went in for my consultation with the doctor, I cried for two hours. I didn't stop crying until I left his office. It was a good thing that my husband was with me, because I didn't hear a thing the doctor said after he mentioned surgery. The first thing I wanted to know is if I can still snowmobile. For, if the doctor told me that I would not be able to do that, dance, or enjoy our boat, I would never have agreed to have surgery. I would rather be active and enjoy my life *until* I have problems.

My X-rays revealed a very rigid spine. In fact, the doctor felt he could only reduce my curve from 95 degrees to about 85 degrees. Right now, I am adjusting to this halo-traction. All the while I kept thinking how I'm doing this because I want to be able to continue all that I love to do. I want to be able to enjoy retirement with my husband which will be in about nine years. We like to do things together. I give credit to him for my growing up and maturing with him. He is so supportive to me.

My biggest hope is that this surgery will stop the progression and any future problems. Since I really didn't have any problems to start with, I hope that none will start. Just from the traction alone, I can feel the difference in the middle of my back. I am sure that things will be even better than I've been told."

MARGARET-ANN

Born: 1938

"I cannot explain the sense of relief that came over me when my surgeon told me he thought surgery would correct some of my physical deformity. Prior to this, I was only hoping for the relief from pain."

Margaret-Ann was born in 1938 and had a spinal fusion at the age of 43. Her scoliosis was detected at the age of 13. As a child her only treatment was exercise because as the doctor told her parents then, "If she were my child, I would leave her alone unless it gives her trouble. Spinal surgery is too risky."

"It was because of pain that I sought medical help. I had not seen a doctor about my back since I was a teenager. The orthopedic surgeon in my hometown referred me to a specialist who treated only spinal deformities. On February 5, 1981, I had Zielke instrumentation and on March 26, 1981, I had Harrington Rods inserted with a spinal fusion. I cannot explain the sense of relief that came over me when my surgeon told me he thought surgery would correct some of my physical deformity. Prior to this, I was only hoping for the relief from pain. I was elated after surgery when my husband reported to me that my back looked almost normal.

My husband and I and our two daughters enjoy spending two weeks each summer at the beach, taking long walks and looking for shells and shark's teeth. Gradually, however, I had to shorten my walks and eventually stop them because of the pain in my leg. This summer, my husband thought it would be best to cancel our beach vacation because I'll be wearing a cast. I want to go because I need to prove to myself that I can still walk along the beach without pain returning to my leg.

My father had a deformed right arm and hand. Although he could use it to some extent, he could not use his hand as most people do. This never stopped him! He pitched college baseball in his younger years, and I always felt he could do everything. Since he had a positive attitude about himself, I believe it helped me develop the same about myself. Although my curve was severe, 90 degrees, I never let the physical deformity bother me. The only negative comment I remember, came from a small child who said, 'Margaret-Ann, why don't you stand up straight? You are so crooked.'

Up until about five years ago, scoliosis did not affect my activities. I graduated college, got married, worked two years at a television station as a secretary, and then retired to raise a family. Since then, I have done housework and yardwork including sprigging, mowing, raking, etc. I have had some difficulty since my surgery. The reason is that I just don't know how to ask for help. Although my friends, neighbors, and family wanted to do something, it was up to me to tell them what was needed to be done. Many times I have felt like I would scream if one more person said, 'Let me get that for you, or let me do that for you.'

Before my surgery, one hip was definitely higher than the other and the left side of my back protruded. My wardrobe consisted mainly of shifts and other blouses to wear with slacks. I don't believe it will be quite as noticeable now that I have had the surgery. I wear a bathing suit, but always choose one that completely covers me. We have a summer cottage on the lake, so wearing a bathing suit has always been part of my life. I have never been able to swim, however. I don't have enough strength in my legs to kick hard enough. When I kick, my legs gradually sink to the bottom. It may be attributed to my low curve.

Before my surgery, I wanted to talk to someone about the procedure and recuperation period. Shortly before I was scheduled for surgery, I received a letter from a young girl, age 23, who had a spinal fusion by the same doctor. She told me of her growing inches, driving the car and running household chores with a body cast. She and her husband visited me often while I was in the hospital. That helped because I was quite a distance from my home and family. Only my husband stayed nearby. Their visits meant a great deal to me."

UPDATE:
"Now that my surgery is over with, I never realized just how self-conscious I was about my misshapen body. I guess I was just too busy to think much about it. The first thing I did after the cast was removed was look at my back to see if my husband was telling me the truth about both sides of my back being practically the same. Until this day, when I shower, I find myself running the cloth down my back and thinking how lucky I am. Maybe I'm just reassuring myself that the hump is not returning.

I truly valued talking with people who had been through this surgery. Although the surgeon was the one to give the information and perform the surgery, he never had the operation. There is nothing like talking with someone who has had the experience first hand."

KIM

Born: 1949

"I am so happy now that I've had surgery. I feel that now I can walk tall into a room. I want to say to people, "Hey, look at me, look how good I look."

Kim was born in 1949. When it was determined at age 13 that she had scoliosis, the doctor recommended that the possibility of surgery existed. He explained that the first procedure would be to do the upper curve, then at a later date, do the lower curve. He recommended spending a period of six months in a body cast with each surgery and staying out of school for a year. There were no guarantees, however, with the outcome, and paralysis was certainly a risk. When Kim's parents heard *paralysis,* they said, "Forget it!"

"I knew nothing about what was wrong with me other than my back was crooked. I was always led to believe, when I was younger, that there wasn't anything that could be done. I was told that there would be a point in time where I was fully matured and my curve wouldn't get worse.

I didn't really start having problems until I was 35 years old. I was always self-conscious about every part of my body. Although my husband never said anything, I was totally ashamed about the way I looked. My bust faced a different direction than my lower trunk. I just always felt so ugly, that I never wanted to take my clothes off in front of him.

Last spring when I discovered that my curve was progressing, I made an appointment with an orthopedic surgeon. I was in severe pain and was told that I had a pinched nerve. The pain would wake me up in the middle of the night and I would have to get up and walk around. It seemed that after I did that, the pain would subside. My curve was measured as 80 degrees thoracic and 64 degrees lumbar.

The doctor recommended surgery and explained the procedure to me and my husband. There was no doubt in my mind that this was what I wanted. I'll never regret having surgery. I feel it's the best thing I've ever done. My curve after correction measures 39 degrees thoracic and 36 degrees lumbar—a well-balanced curve.

I went into this surgery with such an optimistic outlook. I would tell people that I was looking forward to having this surgery. I was just so anxious and excited that I wanted everyone to know. I feel like I've been offered a new beginning of life. People say to me, 'Kim, you look like you've lost a lot of weight.' But what they really see is a waist. Instead of seeing the ribs sticking out in front and my hip sticking out in back, I am in a straight up and down appearance. I am also an inch taller. Just the other day, my husband commented on my back. He said, 'Your body looks just beautiful.' I know he just can't wait until I get this plastic jacket off for good so he can get right to it and enjoy the new me.

I think that school screening for early detection for scoliosis is the greatest thing that could have come about. My recommendations to a family first finding out that their child has scoliosis would be to keep up with it and don't say that the problem will go away. See a doctor who specializes in scoliosis and follow his recommendation.

I am so happy now that I've had surgery. I feel that now I can walk tall into a room. I want to say to people, 'Hey, look at me, look how good I look.' Sure you take a chance that it might fail, and maybe it won't even be corrected as much as you would like, but surgery can stop the progression. I feel like this surgery is not only a new beginning for me, but it has added years on to my life."

CHAPTER **5**

I Married My Wife for Her Curves! The Spouses Respond

Necessary to completing a more total picture of the emotional end of scoliosis treatment was to include responses from the spouses. They were most willing to share their feelings and anxieties about their spouses treatment.

The responses received were generally supportive. They all appeared eager for their mate to have the surgery, if it was indicated by the attending physician. Improvement in the quality of life was what all felt was the determining factor in surgery. As one husband put it, "I married my wife for her curves!"

Properly fitting clothing, sexual relations, general health and well being, and worry over complications were concerns expressed by the spouses regarding surgery. Each spouse interviewed expressed their support and understanding for their mate.

Another determining factor in the decision to have surgery was pain. "For a year prior to surgery, my wife complained frequently of pain in her lower back and leg. She had very little energy and was periodically depressed. I noticed she required a great deal of sleep. Presently, she is in a body cast, but appears to have a lot more energy even in this state than she did before. I feel that I have been emotionally supportive. I left the decision to have surgery up to my wife, but I gave advice when asked. Together we made the necessary arrangements. I took time off from work and stayed with her during both periods of surgery which were out of state."

Of major concern to the person with scoliosis is self-image and attractiveness. To the spouse, however, good health, well-being, and a pain-free life, was the major concern. "My wife felt unattractive and fat in the body cast, which made her depressed. This didn't affect me because I knew she would be pretty after the cast came off. I was most worried that the surgery wouldn't work and she might be paralyzed. But, I still thought it was worth the risk to alleviate the pain she was experiencing."

No spouse expressed any concern over sexual relationships after the surgery. Mostly, this was the concern of the scoliosis patient. "Scoliosis has not affected my sexual feelings toward my husband. I wish for his sake, his back was straight, but it has no effect on our sex life. I love my husband a great deal and worry more about the surgical complications more than anything else." Another spouse relates: "Once my wife got used to the body cast, our sex life improved markedly. She was very nervous and uptight prior to the operation, but afterwards she relaxed and allowed herself to enjoy our sexual relations."

Often times the spouse felt a sense of loss on how to be helpful in the decision making process. "I was most worried about my wife's ability to come through the surgery without any side complications. Before the surgery, the increasing hump in my wife's back distressed me. I did not discuss it with her because I was afraid to make her self-conscious. At least that was my rationalization. I, too, have a chronic health problem. I figured that both of us would be able to understand and support one another. I am not sure, however, if we were aware of the genetic aspects before we had children. I was concerned, however, about the effects of pregnancy on her back and encouraged her to go to a doctor for consultation. We now tend to believe that her pregnancies caused her curvature to increase. After our second child was born, I felt that her curvature was much more pronounced. With regard to friendships, my wife's personality is such that people do not notice the deformity first. The positive, outgoing personality is what the public notices first. Because of this, I don't think her back is a problem to her in making friends."

Clothing presented a major problem to the scoliosis patient, so the spouses responded this way: "About three years ago we began consulting with a scoliosis specialist about my wife's scoliosis. This was triggered, at least in part, because she had so much trouble getting clothes to fit." Another spouse remarked that she feels her husband is much more critical of what he wears than she. "He limits his clothing choices to things that deemphasize his curvature. There are occasions when the fit of his clothing bothers me and I quietly try to adjust his collar or tie. Regretably, this makes him more self-conscious."

A wife of 52 years makes the following statement about her husband's severe scoliosis. "I was very concerned about his planting shrubs and trees this spring. The pressure he put on a shovel with his feet, I felt, was damaging to his back. But, he says, it doesn't produce pain."

What clearly came through in these interviews, was the love shared between these couples. That had a greater overall effect on the well-being than the actual scoliosis itself. To sum up, "My husband has a fantastic self-image except when it comes to scoliosis. I am used to his handling a lot of jobs around our home and his always being in control of the situation. As the years of marriage go on, it becomes easier to discuss these feelings and problems. I used to be very worried about hurting his feelings or drawing attention to his scoliosis. But, to be quite honest, what really matters is that I love my husband very much."

CHAPTER 6

Update . . . Scoliosis. A Discussion with Iris, Terry, and Stephanie

> *Knowledge of the past is essential and relevant to our ability to understand the present and plan for the future. In order to stop being a victim of the past, one must become enlightened and involved. A positive attitude on the part of the patient constitutes at least half of the recovery from scoliosis treatment.*

In the discussion to follow, I talked with Stephanie and Terry about their surgeries that took place in the 80's as adults. Both are career women, well-informed, and have positive attitudes about the surgery and its outcome. Terry is a registered nurse. As a result of her medical background she insisted on being part of the decision-making process regarding her treatment. Stephanie has a management position with the U.S. Army. Her physician father helped to enlighten her about treatment for scoliosis and maintain a positive attitude.

Both women are single career women whose recollections make it increasingly clear that attitudes have definitely improved on the part of the patient and treatment. These two women explain in detail the steps they took to arrive at their decision to have surgery as an adult.

Terry was born in 1953. Her surgery was scheduled in 1984. Her curve now measures 23 degrees. Stephanie was born in 1950. She is divorced, wore a Milwaukee Brace as a child and had surgery as an adult. Her curve now measures 42 degrees.

A DISCUSSION

TERRY: My scoliosis was not a big problem until I was 29 years old. Pain was limiting my activities. My friends didn't really understand my problem of facing surgery. My family basically was supportive, but I was reluctant to let them know of my very high anxiety level because I didn't want them to worry. Subsequently, I bore the burden of anxiety and fear myself—sometimes not being very pleasant to be around. I've always envied those persons with straight bodies and feel my body is quite unattractive. My biggest problem was deciding on surgery and what surgical procedure was best for my problem. Each consultation averaged about $50.00. It was like talking to a car salesman. Each surgeon wanted to do a different instrumentation and they varied on how many vertebra to fuse. All of this was very confusing. I was off from work for a total of seven months. During that time I was not allowed to work in the hospital in any capacity while wearing a post-surgical brace. I felt fine and could do anything I wanted including painting the house while wearing the brace. I received 13 weeks disability pay which was 80% of my work pay. After that, I had to pay for my own health insurance and borrow money for living expenses. I eventually lost my job in the recovery room and had to be reinterviewed for my current position in labor and delivery.

STEPHANIE: I remember being the only student eliminated from the eighth grade school play because I was wearing a brace. No one in the private school I attended thought this unusual at all. When I cried at home, I remember my father telling me I'd better get used to it. Experiences like that just slowly caused me to crawl into a mental and emotional shell. I consider myself to be in relatively good health. I usually swim several miles a week. I was given no restrictions following surgery except for sky diving, hang gliding, boxing, football or high diving. Other than that, I do everything else I want.

STEPHANIE: My dad was a doctor. I was probably treated in a most advanced manner. He took me all the way to Minnesota every few months from California where we lived. We did that for years. In 1962, I was the first person that I know of that wore a Milwaukee Brace from my part of town.

IRIS: How do both of you feel about your future with scoliosis? Are you worried about it and do you have any particular concerns?

STEPHANIE: No, none.

TERRY: Yes, I think I do have a slight concern because with the fusion I was told that I could expect to have some arthritic changes. I figured that I had nothing to lose because I was going to be crippled by the time I was 40 if I didn't do something; or I was going to take a chance on having some pain or arthritic changes by the time I was 40 even if I had surgery.

IRIS: Stephanie, do you have any resentments about the fact that you had to wear a Milwaukee Brace for many years and then still required surgery?

STEPHANIE: Yes, gee I feel, what a waste of time! But, the doctor I saw told me that the only reason I am so educated is because I have had a massive dosage of treatment. I spent nine years, to be exact, wearing a Milwaukee Brace.

IRIS: Are you satisfied with the treatment you received, and the answers to your questions regarding surgery, from your doctor?

TERRY: As far as surgically, I am very satisfied. The only thing I was concerned with was not being in pain—and I have no pain.

STEPHANIE: Physically, I felt wonderful. As far as the outcome of my curvature, I just wish the numbers were lower. Everybody says I look real good.

IRIS: Do you feel self-conscious about any part of your body due to scoliosis?

STEPHANIE: Yes, the whole thing—my hips, back, the whole thing.

TERRY: Yes, my hips worry me a bit. But they are much better now than they were. The worst part is the lack of lordosis, because my back doesn't have a sway to it.

IRIS: When I had my surgery at the age of 13, I had to lie flat on my back with a body cast that went from the top of my head to my hips for six months. With the next cast that trimmed down the head piece, was another 4 months. I missed a whole year of school and was tutored by an inservice teacher. Personally, I feel that dealing with surgery of any kind is difficult. But, in particular scoliosis surgery involved a dependency and a loss of control. In a sense, we get the feeling of being physically disabled, even if only a temporary condition.

STEPHANIE: That feeling comes from my childhood and is probably the reason I am so independent today. One just utterly hates to be so out of it. There are so many people at my job that carry on about some minor thing. I'll tell them I went through something really major and personally, I think I breezed through it.

IRIS: It must be really difficult to make the decision to have surgery as an adult. It involves so many things like putting your life in order, the thought of temporary disability or loss of income, and so many unknown risks.

TERRY: I lived with my family for two or three months and my sister stayed at my place and paid my rent. Then, when I moved back home I had a friend come and live with me to help pay the rent. My family was very supportive, but I found that whole thing difficult, especially in the hospital. I was always used to taking care of other people and those other people depending on me. Then, suddenly the tables were turned and I was the one who was dependent. Coming back home also presented a problem. Moving in with my parents presented lots of guilt.

STEPHANIE: I had to come home for three weeks, too. I flew on an airplane to California. The doctor said that I couldn't take care of myself and I really wasn't in any position to argue. My mother and father at the time were both very sick—my dad had cancer and my mother other health problems. What a terrible experience. So many things enter into the total picture for recovery.

IRIS: Do you feel that having had to cope with scoliosis and treatment has made you special?

TERRY: I just feel that if I got through that surgery, I can get through anything.

STEPHANIE: That's the same with me. People say that I am real calm in a disaster.

IRIS: Suppose you did not have scoliosis and a cosmetic deformity. How would that have changed your life?

STEPHANIE: Oh, my whole life would be different. If I didn't have scoliosis, I wouldn't be so hung up on career success and would probably be married and have some kids. I was always worried about paying bills first.

TERRY: I don't think anything would have been different except for now I am really interested in a career change. I think because of my experience with scoliosis I might want to do something in the area of orthotics or assisting in scoliosis surgery.

IRIS: Has scoliosis had a positive or negative effect on your self image?

TERRY: I think negative. I'd love to have a straight back. Everytime I see those girls and guys at the beach and just how strong and straight their backs look, I get so envious.

STEPHANIE: Oh, I'm sure it was very negative. But, it has changed lately to being more positive. I feel like the lady who has lost a hundred pounds. I feel proud of it.

IRIS: People do not understand how much trouble those of us with scoliosis have to go through to look good. One of the important things that we, as a support group, can offer is to help people dress better to improve one's self-image. Clothing is very important especially in camouflaging the deformity.

TERRY: I remember the first meeting I went to with my mom. I was in tears. I mean I heard scoliosis referred to as a deformity. That really humiliated me to think that I was deformed. No, people really don't understand.

IRIS: A big drawback with scoliosis is that it occurs during the most vulnerable part of a young person's life—teenage years. Even treatment for a year or two seems like an eternity to a teenager who can't conceptualize the future. They think in terms of right now.

STEPHANIE: That's what the problem is, one needs to be grown up before getting sick. It's very hard to get scoliosis as a kid and learn to deal with it on adult terms.

IRIS: Do you feel that having scoliosis has made you more critical of yourself by proving your limitations or achievements?

STEPHANIE: Absolutely! Who else would be concerned day and night about standing up straight.

IRIS: Unfortunately, our society places a great deal of emphasis on physical appearance. One can't help but become extremely critical when our bodies do not measure up to what society is viewing as normal.

TERRY: Right! It's not like being fat. When you're fat, you do have a chance to lose weight. But, when you have a deformity like scoliosis, you just kind of have to . . .

STEPHANIE: Live with it!

TERRY: Right!

IRIS: Do you feel that your lifetime goals have changed in the past five to ten years? Has scoliosis had an effect on this attitude?

TERRY: Of course my goals have changed, but I think that it is not because of scoliosis, but rather because of my age.

STEPHANIE: Oh, mine have changed completely, but not totally due to scoliosis. Part was due to my divorce. I now see a real rugged future for myself, work wise. My father never expected me to get married. I was just supposed to earn a living and face a life of disability. My father also made it very clear to me that I was never going to get anything other people had and I just had better wake up and use my brain. So, I never aspired to what the average person has. By that I mean, a home, a family and a husband. That would just have been a gift. I would have been dazzled by it.

IRIS: Do you blame any one particular factor for your being what you are or what you are not?

TERRY: No, I don't think so. I am just so very happy about the whole thing and the outcome. I made all the decisions as an adult and on my own. I am very happy about that.

STEPHANIE: I think the problems in childhood are far more serious than the adults have to face. I may be rather naive about this, but scoliosis has been an asset to my life. Rather than see it as a disability, I think I have developed a lot of inner control over my feelings. I see it at work and in my business dealings with people.

IRIS: What kind of advice would you offer to a parent or child finding out for the first time that they have scoliosis? What are the most significant questions you feel should be addressed?

STEPHANIE: Things are better today than before. I would always tell them that first. Braces look better, they are put on earlier and the results are better.

TERRY: I think about the fact that there is just so much more information available. For example through the Scoliosis Association, Inc. reading materials may be obtained, people are there to talk to, meetings and specialists are available to the public, and in general there is a great deal more public awareness available now than ever before. Years ago this was not even an option. I guess I'm just real happy with what was done to me.

PART III
Getting it Straight

CHAPTER **1**

How to Look for a Spinal Deformity

Most scoliosis does not produce pain in early stages of development. Therefore, it is possible to go unnoticed by the person who has it, the conscientious parent who checks regularly for health problems, and sometimes the doctor. All children should be checked by either a school nurse, a teacher, a parent, or a doctor with a similar procedure as described below. If a problem exists, consult with your family doctor or orthopedic surgeon.

Have the child remove his/her shirt and stand straight up with arms dangling loosely down. Sit in a chair with the child standing in front of you but facing away and again facing you. (See figure 5 and figure 6.)

1. Does the child look balanced and straight?
2. Is one shoulder higher than the other?
3. Is there an unevenness of the wings of the shoulder blades?
4. Is one hip higher than the other?
5. Is there a greater distance between the arm and the body on one side when the arms are hanging loosely?
6. Is the waistline symmetrical?
7. Is the spine straight to sight and touch from the neck to the buttocks?
8. Is the child leaning toward one side or the other?

In the forward bending position, have the child bend forward until his/her back is parallel to the floor. Have the palms of each hand touch each other at about knee level.

1. Are there any bulges in the shoulder area?
2. Is there a bulge in the lumbar area near the waist?
3. Do you see "round shoulders" or kyphosis?
4. Do you see a "swayback" or lordosis?

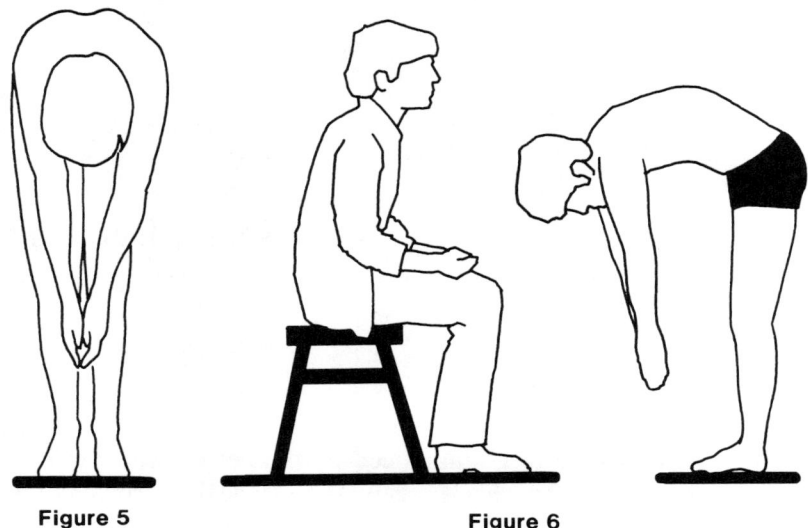

Figure 5. A front view of forward bend.

Figure 6. Subject in forward bend position with screener sitting in chair.

Often times scoliosis is first noticed by clothing that doesn't fit properly—uneven hemlines or pant legs. If scoliosis is present in your family, or your child shows signs of having scoliosis, be sure to have it checked by your family physician or orthopedic surgeon. There is sufficient evidence available through school screening and research to indicate that the key to preventing future problems in adult life is early detection and prompt treatment.

CHAPTER **2**

Postural Exercises for Scoliosis

The exercises listed within are standard back strengthening and posture awareness exercises. They should be done with the assistance of a competent physical therapist or physician who specializes in this training. *It is important to remember that before starting and while engaging in any exercise program, one should consult with a physician concerning specific health needs.*

The purpose of an exercise program is to maintain the proper alignment of the spine while keeping the head in the proper position and preventing any excessive thoracic kyphosis and lumbar lordosis. The goals of a physical therapy program in the treatment of scoliosis is to:

1. improve mobility by identifying and correcting any functional deficiency such as limited *range of motion* or weakness of any of the joints especially when there is an imbalance between the right and left side,
2. improve stability by maintaining the strength of the trunk musculature and strengthening the muscles to maintain the spine in a straightened position,
3. provide patient education with the specific exercise instruction.

To accomplish these goals the exercise programs must be tailored to the patient. This can be done by a competent physical therapist or physician who has specialized training and who is knowledgeable in the biomechanics of scoliosis. The individual exercises are prescribed much like medication for the patient. **If they are prescribed wrong or performed incorrectly, they may not help the condition and quite possibly serve to worsen it.**

Begin slowly and build steadily into a routine. No exercise should cause pain or discomfort. If that should happen, one is either doing it wrong, too vigorously, or is not in good condition for that exercise. Finally, it is important to be consistent in following the exercise program.

ABDOMINAL STRENGTHENING

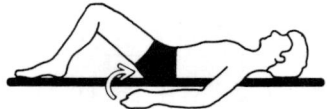

Figure 7

Figure 7. Pelvic tilt supine. Exercise on a firm surface preferably a carpeted floor. Lie on your back and keep both knees bent. Tighten the abdominal muscles and the buttocks by tilting the pelvis slightly backward, flattening the low back into the floor. Hold for a count of ten, *breathing in and out normally.*

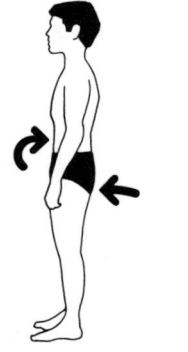

Figure 8

Figure 8. Pelvic tilt standing. Tighten the abdominal muscles and tilt the pelvis while standing. Breathe in and out slowly while holding the pelvic tilt. This exercise can also be done in the sitting position.

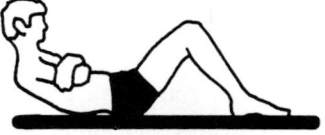

Figure 9

Figure 9. Partial sit-ups. In the same position as the pelvic tilt supine, position arms across shoulders. While doing the pelvic tilt, raise head and shoulders off the surface. Lower slowly. Always do the sit-ups keeping the knees bent and both feet flat.

BACK STRETCHING EXERCISE

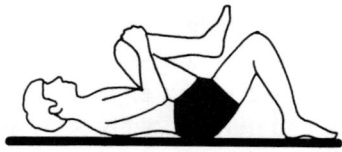

Figure 10

Figure 10. Knees to chest. Lie on your back with both knees bent. Tighten the abdominal muscles then raise one knee toward your chest. Grasp the knee with one hand and relax the abdominals. Gently stretch the back by pulling the knee toward the shoulder. Hold for a count of five. Breathe normally, exhaling as you stretch.

Bring each knee to chest one at a time.

LEG STRENGTHENING EXERCISE

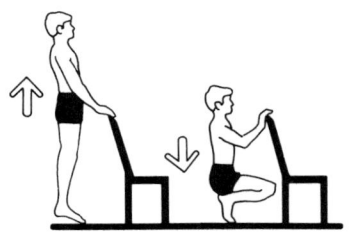

Figure 11. Stand with your feet a comfortable distance apart. Lightly hold onto the back of a chair for balance. Tighten the abdominal muscles and slowly lower the trunk bending only at the hips and knees keeping the trunk straight. Come down and up slowly.

Figure 11

The emphasis on an entire exercise program is to increase posture awareness. With increased posture awareness there is a need to change the behavior of adapting the abnormal postural habit. Once one has learned to correct the posture a conscious effort must continually be made to make the postural adjustment.

The exercises described within are only a partial list that may be used to strengthen and stretch back and abdominal muscles. *Once again, it is important to consult with a physician before engaging in any specific exercise program especially with a specific health concern.*

CHAPTER **3**

Glossary of Scoliosis Terms

Adolescent Scoliosis A spinal curvature discovered between puberty and the completion of skeletal growth.

Adult Scoliosis A spinal curvature existing beyond the age of completion of growth or skeletal maturity. The adult spine is less flexible and thus less reversible or correctable by the elimination of gravity, flexibility, exercises, braces or casting.

Anterior Spine Instrumentation Systems for the Treatment of Scoliosis

Dwyer Instrumentation A. F. Dwyer in 1974 developed an anterior approach to the spine in which discs are removed and the spine is fixed with screws and a flexible cable applied to the vertebral bodies. The advantage is powerful correction of lumbar and thoracolumbar curves.

Zielke Instrumentation Zielke followed in 1977 with an anterior, interbody fixation similar to Dwyer but utilizing a solid rod rather than a flexible cable to gain correction. The advantage is a rigid fixation with good correction of lumbar curves. This system does require post-operative external support with a cast or brace.

Cervico-Thoracic A spinal curvature which has its apex at C7 or T1. A less common curve pattern.

Chronological Age Age determined by birth date.

Compensatory Curve (Secondary) A flexible curve developing to maintain spinal balance or body alignment. This usually develops above or below the major curve in an attempt to maintain the normal body alignment.

Congenital Scoliosis A spinal curvature with which a child is born due to a birth defect or abnormality of the spine.

Double Major Curve Often called "S curve." They are thoracic and lumbar curves existing together, generally occurring in opposite directions. Two structural curves.

Double Thoracic A spinal curvature with a structural upper thoracic curve, a larger more deforming lower thoracic, and a relatively non-structural lumbar curve.

Functional Curve A curve that is non-structural. A flexible curve which can be completely corrected by bending. Functional curves have no structural changes. These curves correct or over correct.

Hyperkyphosis An excessive degree of kyphosis which is abnormal.

Hyperlordosis An excessive degree of lordosis which is abnormal.

Idiopathic Scoliosis A spinal curvature in which the cause is yet unknown, comprising the largest single group of scoliosis patients. There may be many or several causes—very likely an inherited problem with possible sex linkage.

Iliac Crest Apophysis An indicator of bone growth in the hip region determined by an X-ray. As long as an open line is observed on the X-ray and no fusion noted, further spine growth can be expected and more progression of scoliosis is possible.

Infantile Idiopathic A spinal curvature discovered and developing before age 3—not common in the United States.

Juvenile Scoliosis A spinal curvature discovered between age 3 and the onset of puberty—between the ages of three and 14 years.

Kyphosis A forward bending of the thoracic spine. Twenty to forty degrees of kyphosis is considered a normal range.

Lumbar Curve A curve lying mainly in the lumbar spine—lower back curve. A spinal curvature which has its apex from L1 to L4.

Lumbar Lordosis A swayback. A normal curvature in a spine viewed from the side—pathologic when excessive.

Lumbosacral A curvature which has its apex at L5 or below.

Major Curve Designates large curve requiring treatment (e.g. over 20 degrees). Usually structural, it is the largest curve with the greatest angulation.

Minor Curve Small curves, usually not progressive, requiring only observation.

Neuromuscular Scoliosis A spinal curvature due to an abnormality in a muscle function either due to muscle disease, a disorder or anomalies in the nervous system.

Pelvic Obliquity A tilting of the pelvis. This is created by the attempt of the spine to assume balance to the center of gravity.

Posterior Spine Instrumentation Systems for the Treatment of Scoliosis

Harrington Instrumentation Dr. Paul R. Harrington in the late 1950's devised a posterior rod system with distraction applied to the concavity of a scoliotic deformity with compression forces exerted on the convexity. It was the first effective surgical instrumentation for the treatment of scoliosis. Harrington instrumentation is the *gold standard* by which all others must be measured.

Luque Instrumentation Eduardo Luque in 1974 in Mexico City developed a sublaminar wiring to bilateral rods achieving segmental fixation of the spine. The advantage to using this system is greater fixation. However, the disadvantage is greater risk of neurologic injury.

Drummond Spinal Fixation Dennis Drummond in 1984 developed a spinous process wire fixation to a Harrington distraction rod on the concavity of a curve with a Luque rod applied to the convexity. The advantage to this system is superior early stability decreasing the need for an external cast or brace support. There is less risk of neurologic injury with this system.

Cotrel-Dubousset Cotrel and Dubousset in 1984 in France developed a posterior rod and multiple hook system achieving segmental fixation and strong correction of curves. The advantage of this system is good fixation with better correction of rotational deformity. However, the disadvantage is greater risk of neurologic compromise.

Rib Prominence A fullness or prominence of the rib cage caused by rotation of the spine.

Rotation A twisting about the long axis of the spine.

Scoliosis A medical term for the side-to-side curving of the spine causing rotation. A spinal deformity that, when left to progress, could cause heart and lung damage, undesirable appearance with physical and psychological problems, pain, and sometimes early death. Scoliosis is the lateral bending versus a normal spine which is perfectly straight.

Skeletal Age or Bone Age The amount of skeletal maturity compared to that expected at a given age.

Structural Curve A curve with intrinsic stiffness of fixation (rigidity) and is non-flexible. In a structural curve a segment of the spine has a fixed curve that does not correct upon lateral bending or in the supine position.

Thoracic Curve A curve which lies primarily in the thoracic spine (that part of the spine associated with the rib cage). The apex between T2 and T11.

Thoracolumbar Curve A spinal curvature which extends throughout the thoracic and lumbar spine. The apex at T12 or L1.

Vertebral Epiphysis The growth plate on the top and bottom of each vertebral body which gives rise to an increase in vertebra height.

CHAPTER 4

Reference List of Recommended Reading

BOOKS

Barr, Linda. *Nothing Hurts But My Heart.* Willowisp Press, Inc. 1987. Worthington, Ohio (Paperback).

Blount, Walter P., M.D., Moe, John H., M.D. *The Milwaukee Brace.* Second Edition. Williams & Wilkins. Baltimore/London. 1980.

Cailliet, Rene, M.D. *Scoliosis Diagnosis and Management.* F. A. Davis Company. Philadelphia 1975, 1977, 1978.

Delpech, J. M. *De l'Orthomorphie.* "Introduction" 1928 Edition Medicina Rara. Boston-Stuttgart.

Griesse, Rosalie. *The Crooked Shall Be Made Straight.* Atlanta: John Knox Press 1979.

Linde, Shirley. *How to Beat A Bad Back.* New York: Rawson, Wade Publishers. 1980.

Moe, John H., M.D., Winter, Robert B., M.D., Bradford, David S., M.D., Lonstein, John E., M.D. *Scoliosis and Related Spinal Deformities.* W. B. Saunders Co., Philadelphia, London, Toronto 1978.

Nobel, Elizabeth. *Essential Exercises for the Childbearing Years.* A Guide to Health and Comfort Before and After Your Baby is Born. Houghton-Mifflin Co., Boston 1976.

Schommer, Nancy. *Stopping Scoliosis.* Doubleday & Co., Inc. Sept. 1987, Garden City, New York, 11530.

Sohrabi, Louise F. *The Crooked Journey.* Rima Press, 1420 Mound St., Alameda, CA 94501. 1983.

Zorab, P. A. Ed. *Scoliosis and Muscle.* SIMP Research Monograph No. 4 1974. Spastics International Med. Publ. London.

PERIODICALS

Bengtsson, G., Fallstron, K., Jansson, B., and Nachemson, A. "A Psychological and Psychiatric Investigation of the Adjustment of Female Scoliosis Patients." *ACTA Psychiat. Scand.* 1971.

Boegli, Emily and Steele, Mary. "Scoliosis, Spinal Instrumentation and Fusion." *American Journal of Nursing.* Nov. 1968 pp. 2399–2403. Ill.

Bome, Kathleen Black. "Halo Traction" *American Journal of Nursing.* Sept. 1969 pp. 1933–1937. Ill.

Cady, J. W. "Dear Pain . . ." *American Journal of Nursing.* June 1976 pp. 960–961.

Dollins, Constance M. "Scoliosis: Strain on Self-Image." *The Journal of Practical Nursing.* May, 1976, p. 27.

"A Glossary of Scoliosis Terms." *Spine.* Vol. 1 No. 1 March, 1976.

Keim, Hugo. "Scoliosis Can Progress in the Adult." *Orthopaedic Review.* Feb. 1974. pp. 23–28. Ill.

Mills, William J., Jr. "Scoliosis: Disease or Inheritance?" *Alaska Medicine.* Sept. 1966 pp. 53–55.

Raynolds, Nancy. "Teaching Parents Home Care After Surgery For Scoliosis." *American Journal of Nursing.* June 1974, pp. 1090–1092.

Sells, Clifford J., and May, Eleanor A. "Scoliosis Screening In Public Schools." *American Journal of Nursing.* Jan. 1974.

Shifrin, Louis. "Recognizing Scoliosis Early." *American Family Physician.* Dec. 1971 pp. 76–82.

"That Aching Back!" *Time.* Vol. 116 No. 2 July 14, 1980.

Winter, Robert B., M.D. "How to Find A Spinal Deformity Look For It." *Modern Medicine.* May 1, 1975. pp. 38–43.

NEWSLETTERS AND PAMPHLETS

Backtalk. Official Publication published quarterly by The Scoliosis Association, Inc. P.O. Box 51353, Raleigh, NC 27609 (919)846–2639. Included with membership dues.

Fenner, Louise. "When the Spine Curves." Reprinted from Sept. 1984 FDA *Consumer* HHS Publ. No. (FDA) 85–4198. Department of Health and Human Services. FDA, 5600 Fishers Lane, Rockville, MD 20857.

Heckman, Lynn A. Et. Al., *What If You Need An Operation For Scoliosis?* Cleveland: Rainbow Hospital Youth Spine Center, 1974.

Keim, Hugo, M.D. F.A.C.S. "Scoliosis" *Clinical Symposia.* Vol. 30, No. 1, 1978.

SCOLIOSIS RESEARCH SOCIETY

Booklets Available on Scoliosis:
1. Adult Spinal Deformity
2. Scoliosis
3. Scoliosis and Kyphosis

Write to:

SCOLIOSIS RESEARCH SOCIETY
222 South Prospect—Suite 127
Park Ridge, IL 60068
(312)698–1627

Associations and Foundations

NATIONAL SCOLIOSIS FOUNDATION
93 Concord Avenue, P.O. Box 547
Belmont, MA 02178
(617)489–0880
Laura B. Gowen, President

THE SCOLIOSIS ASSOCIATION, INC.
P.O. Box 51353
Raleigh, NC 27609
(919)846–2639
Barbara M. Shulman, President